Ross & Wilson

Self-Assessment in Anatomy and Physiology in Health and Illness

FIRST EDITION

Ross & Wilson

Self-Assessment in Anatomy and Physiology in Health and Illness

ANNE WAUGH, BSc (Hons) MSc CertEd SRN RNT PFHEA
Former Senior Teaching Fellow and Senior Lecturer,
School of Health and Social Care,
Edinburgh Napier University,
Edinburgh, UK

ALLISON GRANT, BSc PhD FHEA
Lecturer, Department of Health and Life Sciences,
Glasgow Caledonian University,
Glasgow, UK

ELSEVIER

Edinburgh   London   New York   Oxford   Philadelphia   St Louis   Sydney   2019

ELSEVIER

Adapted from *MCQs for Ross & Wilson Anatomy and Physiology in Health and Illness* which was produced for Al-Farabi College, Saudi Arabia © 2016 Elsevier Ltd. All rights reserved.
ISBN: 978-0-7020-6972-7 / e-ISBN: 978-0-7020-6985-7

This edition published by Elsevier Ltd, Oxford, UK. All rights reserved.
ISBN: 978-0-7020-7830-9 / e-ISBN: 978-0-7020-7828-6

Notices

Practitioners and researchers must always rely on their own experience and knowledge in evaluating and using any information, methods, compounds or experiments described herein. Because of rapid advances in the medical sciences, in particular, independent verification of diagnoses and drug dosages should be made. To the fullest extent of the law, no responsibility is assumed by Elsevier, authors, editors or contributors for any injury and/or damage to persons or property as a matter of products liability, negligence or otherwise, or from any use or operation of any methods, products, instructions, or ideas contained in the material herein.

Printed in India
Last digit is the print number: 9 8 7 6 5

Content Strategist: Alison Taylor
Content Development Specialist: Kirsty Guest
Project Manager: Louisa Talbott
Design: Christian Bilbow

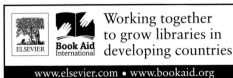

Working together
to grow libraries in
developing countries

ELSEVIER Book Aid International

www.elsevier.com • www.bookaid.org

CONTENTS

PREFACE

Authored and revised by Anne Waugh and Allison Grant, this paperback has been designed to enable you to test your knowledge and understanding of a range of topics fundamental to the study of anatomy and physiology. This quick revision aid is designed to complement the best-selling and well-established *Ross & Wilson Anatomy and Physiology in Health and Illness* publications currently available. Although this book has been prepared as part of the *Ross and Wilson* stable, its scope and level will facilitate anatomy and physiology revision across a wide range of health profession programmes, and will effectively support your study teamed with any standard textbook.

Reflecting the clear structure and systematic approach seen in *Ross & Wilson Anatomy and Physiology in Health and Illness*, each chapter presents a range of multiple choice questions – the number of which broadly reflects the weighting and importance of the topic – designed to facilitate quick review and self-test in key areas of anatomy and physiology. The answers are provided at the end of the book and not only provide an explanation of the correct response, but also the page reference in *Ross & Wilson Anatomy and Physiology in Health and Illness* 13E, where more information on the subject can be found.

We hope that the portable nature of this book will mean that you will not only be able to use it during formal revision settings but also, perhaps, while travelling or on placement. You could also use the material with your colleagues, and revise and test yourselves in study groups.

However and whenever you chose to use the MCQs, we wish you every success with your studies and the best of luck in whatever profession you have chosen!

Anne Waugh and Allison Grant, 2018

CHAPTER 1

Anatomy and Organisation of the Body

Multiple Choice

1. The study of the structure of the body and the physical relationship between its constituent parts is called:
a. Physiology.
b. Pathology.
c. Anatomy.
d. Pathophysiology.

2. The smallest independent units of living matter are:
a. Tissues.
b. Cells.
c. Organs.
d. Systems.

3. Which of the following is principally involved in internal communication within the body?
a. The special senses.
b. The respiratory system.
c. The reproductive system.
d. The endocrine system.

4. The following are examples of transport systems, EXCEPT:
a. The blood.
b. The lymphatic system.
c. The nervous system.
d. The cardiovascular system.

5. In adults, the volume of blood is approximately:
a. 2–3 L.
b. 7–8 L.
c. 5–6 L.
d. 4–5 L.

6. Blood does NOT contain:
a. Plasma.
b. Chromosomes.
c. Platelets.
d. Erythrocytes.

7. Which of the following cells are NOT seen in blood?
   a. Erythrocytes.
   b. Leukocytes.
   c. Thrombocytes.
   d. Adipocytes.

8. Red blood cells:
   a. Transport oxygen and carbon dioxide.
   b. Protect the body against infection.
   c. Assist in blood clotting.
   d. Are larger than white blood cells.

9. Which of the following are NOT blood vessels?
   a. Lymphatics.
   b. Arteries.
   c. Veins.
   d. Capillaries.

10. Capillaries:
    a. Have walls that are only two or three cells thick.
    b. Are the only blood vessels where exchange of substances between the blood and body tissues can take place.
    c. Are part of the lymphatic system.
    d. Carry blood towards the heart.

11. The pulmonary circulation:
    a. Transports blood to and from the lungs.
    b. Transports blood to and from cells in all parts of the body except the lungs.
    c. Transports lymph to the point where it rejoins the bloodstream near the heart.
    d. Transports lymph to and from the lungs.

12. The heart:
    a. Is a muscular sac with four chambers.
    b. Receives blood returning from the body through the arteries.
    c. Beats between 90 and 100 times per minute at rest.
    d. Muscle is under conscious (voluntary) control.

13. In the lymphatic system:
    a. Afferent and efferent lymph vessels are linked by lymphatic capillaries.
    b. The pores in the walls of lymph capillaries are smaller than those of blood capillaries.
    c. Lymph nodes filter lymph, removing microbes and other materials.
    d. There are sites for formation and maturation of erythrocytes.

14. Fast, involuntary and usually protective motor responses to specific stimuli are called:
    a. Motor actions.
    b. Reflex actions.
    c. Nerve impulses.
    d. Feedback actions.

15. Which of the following is NOT one of the special senses?
    a. Smell.
    b. Sight.
    c. Pain.
    d. Balance.

16. In the endocrine system:
   a. A number of glands, situated in different parts of body, are linked by endocrine vessels.
   b. Changes in blood hormone levels are generally controlled by positive feedback mechanisms.
   c. Endocrine glands synthesise and secrete hormones.
   d. The responses that control body functions are slower but less precise than those of the nervous system.

17. An accessory organ of the digestive system is the:
   a. Liver.
   b. Rectum.
   c. Pharynx.
   d. Stomach.

18. Vital gas exchange between the lungs and blood takes place in the:
   a. Trachea.
   b. Bronchi and bronchioles.
   c. Bronchi.
   d. Alveoli.

19. The sum total of the chemical activity in the body is called:
   a. Anabolism.
   b. Catabolism.
   c. Metabolism.
   d. Homeostasis.

20. A zygote is:
   a. A fertilised egg.
   b. A female gamete.
   c. A male gamete.
   d. Another term for a fetus.

21. Structures nearer to the midline are described as:
   a. Anterior.
   b. Medial.
   c. Lateral.
   d. Superior.

22. The term brachial refers to the:
   a. Head.
   b. Navel.
   c. Arm.
   d. Leg.

23. Which of the following is NOT a part of the axial skeleton?
   a. The skull.
   b. The vertebral column.
   c. The ribs.
   d. The shoulder girdle.

24. The only movable bone of the skull is the:
   a. Frontal bone.
   b. Maxilla.
   c. Mandible.
   d. Temporal bone.

25. The intercostal muscles are attached to:
   a. The skull.
   b. The vertebral column.
   c. The thoracic cage.
   d. The shoulder girdle.

26. The space between the lungs is called:
   a. The peritoneum.
   b. The mediastinum.
   c. The pericardium.
   d. The thoracic cavity.

27. Which of the following is NOT a region of the abdominal cavity?
   a. The hypogastric region.
   b. The left iliac fossa.
   c. The hypochondriac region.
   d. The diaphragm.

28. The nature of a disease process and its effect on normal body function is called:
   a. Aetiology.
   b. Pathogenesis.
   c. Complications.
   d. Prognosis.

29. A tissue response to any kind of tissue damage is known as:
   a. Inflammation.
   b. An abnormal immune response.
   c. Thrombosis.
   d. Degeneration.

30. A condition that results from healthcare intervention is called:
   a. Acquired.
   b. Communicable.
   c. Iatrogenic.
   d. A syndrome.

CHAPTER 2

Physiological Chemistry and Processes

Multiple Choice

1. In chemistry:
   a. Elements contain more than one kind of atom.
   b. Atoms of the same type combine to form compounds.
   c. Water is a compound, not an element.
   d. The body is composed almost entirely of only eight types of atom.

2. Within the atomic nucleus are:
   a. Negatively charged electrons, which give the nucleus mass.
   b. Protons; the number of protons is called the atomic number.
   c. Neutrons, electrons and protons, the sum of which is called the atomic weight.
   d. Protons and electrons, the sum of which is called the atomic weight.

3. The atom with eight neutrons, eight protons and eight electrons is:
   a. Oxygen.
   b. Sodium.
   c. Potassium.
   d. Carbon.

4. Chlorine has an atomic weight of 35.5, which is not a whole number because it is the average of how many isotopes of chlorine?
   a. Three.
   b. Six.
   c. Four.
   d. Two.

5. A stable atom could have:
   a. One electron shell, with two electrons in it.
   b. Two electron shells, with two electrons in the inner shell and six in the outer shell.
   c. Three electron shells, with eight electrons in each.
   d. Two electron shells, with eight electrons in each.

6. In a sodium chloride molecule:
   a. The bond between the atoms is covalent.
   b. There are two atoms of sodium and one of chlorine.
   c. The molecule dissolves in water to give positively charged sodium ions.
   d. The bond linking the atoms is strong and very stable.

7. The normal plasma sodium concentration is:
   a. 10–18 mmol/L.
   b. 135–143 mmol/L.
   c. 31–35 mmol/L.
   d. 56–66 mmol/L.

8. Which of the following body fluids is alkaline?
   a. Breast milk.
   b. Gastric juice.
   c. Saliva.
   d. Blood.

9. Which of the following usually contains carbon, oxygen and hydrogen in a 1:1:2 ratio?
   a. Carbohydrates.
   b. Proteins.
   c. Lipids.
   d. Nucleotides.

10. ATP (adenosine triphosphate) contains which of the following?
    a. Deoxyribose sugar, a phospholipid and a base.
    b. Ribose sugar, a base and three phosphate groups.
    c. Three phosphorylated sugars, a base and the amino acid adenosine.
    d. Three fatty acids, ribose sugar and a phospholipid backbone.

11. Phospholipids:
    a. Provide structural support for DNA in the cell nucleus.
    b. Are stored as fat in adipose tissue.
    c. Assemble in a double layer to form cell membranes.
    d. Pad and insulate body organs.

12. What is the role of ATP in cellular energy metabolism?
    a. ATP is broken down in the presence of oxygen to release energy.
    b. ATP is synthesised by enzymes in the mitochondria, which convert it to ADP by adding on one phosphate group.
    c. When ATP is broken down, it releases oxygen for cellular energy.
    d. Release of energy from cellular metabolism is used to synthesise ATP, which stores this energy until it is required.

13. An anabolic reaction is one where:
    a. A substrate is broken down into two reactants by an enzyme.
    b. Two or more substrates are combined by an enzyme to form a larger product.
    c. The reaction rate is slowed to a manageable speed by the action of an enzyme.
    d. The active site on an enzyme is used to split a reactant into two or more substrates.

14. Homeostasis is defined as:
    a. The ability of body systems in general to resist or reverse change in their environment or activity.
    b. The constantly changing composition of the cellular environment.
    c. The ability of the body to tolerate non-physiological internal environments, such as low gastric pH or low pH and increased heat production in exercising muscles.
    d. The constant, involuntary adjustments made to posture, balance and movement by the autonomic nervous system.

15. Which of the following is controlled by a positive feedback mechanism?
   a. Blood pressure.
   b. Blood volume.
   c. Blood clotting.
   d. Red blood cell numbers.

16. Which of the following is a negative feedback response to a rise in body temperature?
   a. Increased blood pressure.
   b. Fever.
   c. Sweating.
   d. Vasoconstriction of blood vessels in the skin.

17. Which of the following statements applies to osmosis?
   a. It requires energy.
   b. It refers specifically to movement of water and water-soluble molecules.
   c. It occurs across the cell membrane until equilibrium is reached.
   d. It can transfer molecules up a concentration gradient.

18. Which of the following statements applies to diffusion?
   a. It requires no energy.
   b. It always takes place across a semipermeable membrane.
   c. It occurs freely for all molecules across the cell membrane until equilibrium is reached.
   d. It can transfer molecules up a concentration gradient.

19. On average, in a healthy adult, what proportion of body weight is represented by intracellular water?
   a. 8%.
   b. 18%.
   c. 28%.
   d. 38%.

20. The sodium-potassium pump:
   a. Keeps intracellular sodium high and extracellular potassium low.
   b. Keeps intracellular sodium low and extracellular potassium high.
   c. Blocks the movement of potassium and sodium into the cell.
   d. Blocks the movement of potassium and sodium out of the cell.

CHAPTER 3

Cells and Tissues

Multiple Choice

1. The plasma membrane consists of:
   a. A monolayer of phospholipids with the hydrophilic heads facing outwards.
   b. A monolayer of phospholipids with the hydrophobic heads facing outwards.
   c. A bilayer of phospholipids with the hydrophilic heads facing outwards.
   d. A bilayer of phospholipids with the hydrophobic heads facing outwards.

2. Branched carbohydrate molecules attached to some cell membrane surface proteins:
   a. Form receptors (recognition sites) for hormones and other chemicals.
   b. Provide the cell with its immunological identity.
   c. Form transmembrane channels.
   d. Act as enzymes.

3. The plasma membrane is:
   a. Nonpermeable.
   b. Selectively permeable.
   c. Fully permeable.
   d. None of the above.

4. Which membrane transport mechanism uses energy for movement of substances?
   a. The sodium-potassium pump.
   b. Osmosis.
   c. Facilitated diffusion.
   d. Diffusion.

5. Transport of large particles across cell membrane takes place by:
   a. Facilitated diffusion.
   b. Diffusion.
   c. Osmosis
   d. Phagocytosis.

6. Which cells do NOT have nuclei?
   a. Skeletal muscle fibres.
   b. Red blood cells.
   c. White blood cells.
   d. Columnar epithelial cells.

7. Deoxyribonucleic acid (DNA) within a non-dividing cell is called:
   a. A chromosome.
   b. A chromatid.
   c. Chromatin.
   d. The nucleolus.

8. The largest organelle is:
   a. The mitochondrion.
   b. The nucleus.
   c. The ribosome.
   d. The lysosome.

9. Which of the following is a function of smooth endoplasmic reticulum?
   a. Synthesis of lipids and steroid hormones.
   b. Synthesis of proteins.
   c. Synthesis of carbohydrates.
   d. Synthesis of DNA.

10. Which of the following is non-membranous?
   a. Smooth endoplasmic reticulum.
   b. The Golgi apparatus.
   c. Lysosomes.
   d. The centrosome.

11. Single, long, whip-like cell projections containing microtubules are called:
   a. The cytoskeleton.
   b. Flagella.
   c. Microvilli.
   d. Cilia.

12. The period between two cell divisions is known as:
   a. Mitosis.
   b. Meiosis.
   c. The cell cycle.
   d. Interphase.

13. Which of the following is NOT a part of interphase?
   a. G_1 phase.
   b. G_0 phase.
   c. S phase.
   d. G_2 phase.

14. In mitosis, the mitotic spindle appears in:
   a. Prophase.
   b. Metaphase.
   c. Anaphase.
   d. Telophase.

15. Squamous (pavement) epithelium lines:
   a. The trachea.
   b. The stomach.
   c. The bladder.
   d. The heart (endocardium).

16. The type of epithelium found on dry surfaces subjected to wear and tear is:
   a. Columnar epithelium.
   b. Keratinised stratified squamous epithelium.
   c. Nonkeratinised stratified squamous epithelium.
   d. Transitional epithelium.

17. Transitional epithelium is found:
   a. Covering bones.
   b. Forming the conjunctiva of the eyes.
   c. Lining the bladder.
   d. In the middle layer of the heart.

18. Which cell types are NOT found in connective tissue?
   a. Fibroblasts.
   b. Fat cells.
   c. Leukocytes.
   d. Erythrocytes.

19. The connective tissue found in lymph nodes and all lymphatic organs is:
   a. Reticular.
   b. Fibrous.
   c. Elastic.
   d. Elastic fibrocartilage.

20. Which of the following is a part of the monocyte-macrophage (mononuclear phagocyte) defence system?
   a. Kupffer cells in liver sinusoids.
   b. Sinus-lining cells in lymph nodes and the spleen.
   c. Microglial cells in the brain.
   d. All of the above.

21. Which tissue is found within the intervertebral discs?
   a. Hyaline cartilage.
   b. Elastic fibrocartilage.
   c. Fibrocartilage.
   d. Fibrous tissue.

22. Automaticity is a property of:
   a. Smooth muscle.
   b. Skeletal muscle.
   c. Neurones.
   d. Glial cells.

23. Which of the following tissues can regenerate?
   a. Neurones.
   b. Cuboidal epithelium.
   c. Skeletal muscle.
   d. All of the above.

24. An epithelial membrane is found in:
   a. Synovial joints.
   b. The peritoneum lining the thoracic cavity and surrounding the lungs.
   c. The pleura lining the abdominal cavity and surrounding the abdominal organs.
   d. The pericardium lining the pericardial cavity and surrounding the heart.

25. Exocrine glands:
   a. Are made from connective tissue.
   b. Release their secretions into the bloodstream.
   c. Are classified as simple or compound (branching).
   d. Secrete hormones.

26. Genetically programmed death of cells at the end of their lifespan is known as:
   a. Hyperplasia.
   b. Hypertrophy.
   c. Necrosis.
   d. Apoptosis.

27. A tumour arising from glandular tissue is a(n):
   a. Sarcoma.
   b. Adenoma.
   c. Myoma.
   d. Osteoma.

28. A carcinogen:
   a. Induces a variable latent period between exposure and signs of malignancy.
   b. Irreversibly damages cellular DNA.
   c. Can be a virus.
   d. All of the above.

29. Benign tumours:
   a. Typically have poorly differentiated cells.
   b. May spread locally.
   c. Are usually encapsulated.
   d. Are associated with metastases (secondary tumours).

30. When malignant breast tumours metastasise, this is typically to the:
   a. Adrenal glands.
   b. Liver.
   c. Pelvic bones.
   d. Vertebrae, brain and bones.

CHAPTER 4

The Blood

Multiple Choice

1. What proportion of whole blood is normally represented by blood plasma?
a. 35%.
b. 45%.
c. 55%.
d. 65%.

2. Of the following, which represents the largest constituent (by volume) of plasma?
a. Glucose.
b. Plasma proteins.
c. Waste products.
d. Electrolytes.

3. Which of the following is an albumin?
a. Transferrin.
b. Thyroglobulin.
c. Fibrinogen.
d. Immunoglobulin.

4. Which of the following is the best definition of anaemia?
a. The inability of the blood to carry enough oxygen to meet the body's needs.
b. Reduced haemoglobin content in circulating red blood cells.
c. A reduced number of circulating red blood cells.
d. Inadequate iron levels in the blood, resulting in small and pale red blood cells.

5. Which of the following terms means production of blood cells?
a. Erythropoiesis.
b. Haemosynthesis.
c. Leukocytosis.
d. Haemopoiesis.

6. Which of the following is characteristic of erythrocyte structure?
a. They are biconcave discs, meaning the central portion is thicker than the outer portion.
b. They contain very few organelles, to make room for haemoglobin, and the nucleus is smaller than average.
c. Their average diameter is about 7 μm, and their flattened shape allows them to stack in piles for smooth flow.
d. Their membranes are flexible, allowing them to deform as they exit the bloodstream to take oxygen to the tissues.

7. How many haemoglobin molecules does an average red blood cell contain?
   a. 280 million.
   b. 280 thousand.
   c. 2.8 million.
   d. 28 million.

8. Oxyhaemoglobin readily releases its oxygen under all of the following conditions, EXCEPT:
   a. Low tissue pH.
   b. Low tissue oxygen levels.
   c. Low tissue temperature.
   d. High tissue carbon dioxide levels.

9. Which of the following statements describing the life cycle of erythrocytes is true?
   a. Erythropoiesis takes about 27 days.
   b. Erythrocytes are released into the circulation as immature reticulocytes.
   c. Dietary folic acid and vitamin C are required for erythrocyte synthesis.
   d. In adults, erythropoiesis takes place mainly in the marrow cavities of long bones.

10. Which term refers to the weight of haemoglobin in 100 mL of red cells?
    a. Mean cell haemoglobin concentration (MCHC).
    b. Mean cell haemoglobin (MCH).
    c. Mean cell volume (MCV).
    d. Haematocrit.

11. Which of the following is true of erythropoietin?
    a. This hormone acts on the spleen to increase red blood cell breakdown.
    b. In erythropoietin deficiency, the blood becomes viscous and more likely to clot.
    c. Erythropoietin is released by the bone marrow to stimulate red blood cell production.
    d. The main stimulus for erythropoietin release is hypoxia, and its levels are controlled by a negative feedback mechanism.

12. In the blood of someone with blood group O:
    a. Erythrocytes display O type antigens and there are anti-A and anti-B antibodies in the plasma.
    b. Erythrocytes display A and B type antigens, and there are no anti-A nor anti-B antibodies in the plasma.
    c. Erythrocytes display neither A nor B type antigens, and there are anti-A and anti-B antibodies in the plasma.
    d. Erythrocytes display O type antigens, and there are no anti-A nor anti-B antibodies in the plasma.

13. Which is the best explanation for why an individual with blood group A will suffer a transfusion reaction if given blood group B?
    a. The recipient has type A antigens on their erythrocytes, which will react with the anti-A antibodies of blood group B.
    b. The recipient produces anti-B antibodies, which will react with the B type antigens on the donor erythrocytes.
    c. The donated blood contains anti-B antibodies, which will react with the anti-A antibodies produced by the recipient.
    d. The donated blood contains anti-A antibodies, which will react with the A type antigens on the recipient's erythrocytes.

14. Granulocytes arise from which precursor cell type?
   a. Megakaryoblast.
   b. Monoblast.
   c. Lymphoblast.
   d. Myeloblast.

15. Mast cells, which are found in the tissues, are similar to which type of white blood cell?
   a. Neutrophil.
   b. Basophil.
   c. Eosinophil.
   d. Monocyte.

16. Which of the following types of white blood cell is first on the scene in an inflammatory response?
   a. Neutrophil.
   b. Basophil.
   c. Eosinophil.
   d. Monocyte.

17. Which of the following white blood cells transforms into a macrophage?
   a. Neutrophil.
   b. Basophil.
   c. Eosinophil.
   d. Monocyte.

18. Lysosomes in phagocytes:
   a. Contain destructive enzymes.
   b. Are responsible for amoeboid motion.
   c. Produce antibodies.
   d. Recognise and target foreign antigens.

19. Kupffer cells:
   a. Are macrophages found in joints.
   b. Are part of the mononuclear phagocyte system.
   c. Are small and mobile.
   d. Are the shortest-lived type of defence cell.

20. Which of the following statements regarding leukaemia is FALSE?
   a. Exposure to ionising radiation is a risk factor, but there is no known genetic predisposition.
   b. The development of anaemia is a recognised feature of the disease.
   c. The increased predisposition to clotting associated with leukaemia increases the risk of stroke and other thrombotic events.
   d. In acute lymphoblastic leukaemia, children have a much better prognosis than adults.

21. Deficiency of which vitamin directly causes impaired clotting?
   a. Vitamin B_{12}.
   b. Vitamin B_1.
   c. Vitamin K.
   d. Vitamin E.

22. The normal blood platelet count is:
    a. 200,000–350,000/mm^3
    b. 100,000–200,000/mm^3
    c. 400,000–550,000/mm^3
    d. 150,000–250,000/mm^3

23. Which of the following structural features do erythrocytes and platelets have in common?
    a. They are both rich in haemoglobin.
    b. Their average counts in whole blood are in the range 400,000–550,000/mm^3.
    c. They are both produced from megakaryoblasts.
    d. Neither has a nucleus.

24. What is the other name for clotting factor XII?
    a. Christmas factor.
    b. Calcium.
    c. Stable factor.
    d. Hageman factor.

25. Which of the following enzymes is responsible for fibrinolysis?
    a. Thromboplastin.
    b. Plasmin.
    c. Fibrin.
    d. Thrombin.

26. Which of the following factors is NOT involved in the final common pathway of clotting?
    a. Thromboplastin.
    b. Prothrombin.
    c. Fibrinogen.
    d. Thrombin.

27. Intrinsic factor is essential for the production of:
    a. Platelets.
    b. Erythrocytes.
    c. Granulocytes.
    d. Agranulocytes.

28. Von Willebrand disease is a(n):
    a. Clotting disorder caused by deficiency of clotting factor VIII.
    b. Immunodeficiency disorder caused by a failure of leukocyte maturation.
    c. Form of anaemia associated with undersized erythrocytes.
    d. Increased risk of thrombus formation due to overactivation of the clotting cascade.

29. What is heparin?
    a. A clotting factor (also called proaccelerin).
    b. An anticoagulant released from mast cells along with histamine.
    c. An inflammatory mediator released from macrophages.
    d. The main constituent of haemoglobin.

30. The Rhesus protein is:
    a. A clotting factor (also called labile factor).
    b. An inflammatory mediator released from macrophages.
    c. A protein sometimes found on the erythrocyte cell membrane.
    d. Essential for the production of all blood cells in red bone marrow.

CHAPTER 5

The Cardiovascular System

Multiple Choice

1. Which of the following applies only to the structure of the venous wall, and not to both arteries and veins?
a. It is composed of three layers of tissue.
b. The inner layer is called the tunica intima.
c. The endothelium covers the valves built into the vessel wall.
d. The outer layer, the tunica adventitia, is fibrous for protection.

2. An artery that provides the only blood supply to a tissue is called a(n):
a. End artery.
b. Anastomotic artery.
c. Shunt.
d. Arteriole.

3. Why does blood from the hepatic portal vein flow through the liver in sinusoids rather than in conventional capillaries?
a. Their leaky walls allow bile and other enzymes to be secreted into the blood.
b. Their large diameter ensures that blood flow is speeded up to prevent pooling and oedema.
c. Their leaky walls allow the liver cells to extract glucose and other products of digestion efficiently.
d. Their large diameter ensures that red blood cells can deliver increased amounts of oxygen to the metabolically active liver cells.

4. Which of the following is described as a resistance vessel?
a. The aorta.
b. An arteriole.
c. A capillary.
d. A vein.

5. Which of the following statements is true of the capillary?
a. Its wall has a single layer of endothelial cells overlying a thin layer of smooth muscle.
b. Red blood cells do not normally pass through the capillary wall.
c. Plasma proteins exchange freely across the capillary wall.
d. The smallest capillaries have an average diameter of about 20 microns.

6. Roughly how much tissue fluid is drained away every day in lymph vessels?
a. 3 L.
b. 8 L.
c. 13 L.
d. 18 L.

7. Exchange of substances in the tissues is determined by the opposing forces across the capillary wall. Which of the following is true?
   a. Hydrostatic pressure at the arterial end of the capillary is about 5 kPa, and at the venous end this increases to 7 kPa.
   b. Osmotic pressure pulls fluid into the bloodstream and is the main reason why hydrostatic pressure increases as blood flows through the capillary.
   c. Hydrostatic pressure, also referred to as blood pressure, is due mainly to the presence of plasma proteins in the blood.
   d. Osmotic pressure remains the same, at about 3 kPa, as blood flows from the arterial end to the venous end of the capillary.

8. The name given to excess fluid in the tissue spaces is:
   a. Lymph.
   b. Oedema.
   c. Interstitial fluid.
   d. Tissue fluid.

9. The base of the heart is associated with which structure?
   a. The diaphragm.
   b. The 5th costal cartilage.
   c. The xiphoid sternum.
   d. The origin of the aorta.

10. The mediastinum contains:
    a. The diaphragm.
    b. The lungs.
    c. The heart.
    d. The sternum.

11. Which of the following is true of the myocardium?
    a. The cells are unbranched and linked by intercalated discs.
    b. Each muscle cell is individually supplied by a separate nerve fibre.
    c. It contains a network of specialised conducting fibres called sinoatrial fibres.
    d. It is the thickest layer of the heart wall and secretes atrial natriuretic peptide (ANP).

12. The visceral pericardium:
    a. Secretes pleural fluid.
    b. Is firmly attached to the myocardium.
    c. Lines the heart chambers.
    d. Is a fibrous, protective layer.

13. The atrioventricular valves:
    a. Are secured to the interior of the ventricular walls with chordae tendinae.
    b. Conduct electrical impulses between the atria and the ventricles.
    c. Both have three cusps, or flaps.
    d. Are closed during the P wave on the ECG.

14. Narrowing of an atrioventricular valve is called:
    a. Incompetence.
    b. Regurgitation.
    c. Stenosis.
    d. Murmurs.

15. The sinoatrial node lies:
   a. At the origin of the aorta.
   b. In the interventricular septum.
   c. Close to the opening of the superior vena cava.
   d. Immediately above the right atrioventricular valve.

16. What proportion of the left ventricular stroke volume passes into the coronary arteries to supply the myocardium?
   a. 25%.
   b. 15%.
   c. 5%.
   d. 20%.

17. What is the average heart rate in a healthy adult?
   a. 40–60 beats per minute (bpm).
   b. 60–80 bpm.
   c. 80–100 bpm.
   d. 100–120 bpm.

18. What is the definition of sinus tachycardia?
   a. Heart rate over 100 bpm but normal rhythm.
   b. Heart rate over 120 bpm but normal rhythm.
   c. Heart rate over 100 bpm but with an identified ECG abnormality.
   d. Heart rate over 120 bpm with an intermittent ECG abnormality.

19. The atrioventricular node:
   a. Sets the normal heart rate.
   b. Generates electrical signals, but at a faster rate than the sinoatrial node.
   c. Controls blood flow between the atria and the ventricles.
   d. Acts as the heart's secondary pacemaker.

20. Which stage of the cardiac cycle normally lasts the longest?
   a. Complete cardiac diastole.
   b. Ventricular contraction.
   c. Atrial systole.
   d. Atrial contraction.

21. The first heart sound, 'lub', corresponds to:
   a. Closure of the aortic valve.
   b. Opening of the pulmonary valve.
   c. Closure of the atrioventricular valves.
   d. Ejection of blood into the aorta.

22. Which is the correct order in which the electrical signal in the heart triggers contraction?
   a. Sinoatrial node, atrioventricular node, Purkinje fibres, right bundle branch.
   b. Atrioventricular node, bundle of His, left bundle branch, Purkinje fibres.
   c. Sinoatrial node, atrial myocardium, right bundle branch, atrioventricular node.
   d. Atrioventricular node, atrial myocardium, left bundle branch, Purkinje fibres.

23. Which of the following is generated by ventricular excitation on an ECG recording?
   a. P wave.
   b. T wave.
   c. P-R interval.
   d. QRS complex.

24. What is heart block?
   a. Obstruction of blood flow anywhere within the heart chambers.
   b. Impairment of the pumping action of the heart, e.g., by cardiac tamponade.
   c. Interference with impulse conduction between the atria and the ventricles.
   d. Reduced contractility of the heart muscle, e.g., following myocardial infarction.

25. The systemic blood pressure recorded during ventricular contraction is called the:
   a. Systolic pressure.
   b. Diastolic pressure.
   c. Pulse pressure.
   d. Mean arterial pressure.

26. Which of the following is true of complete cardiac diastole?
   a. The atria are filling but the atrioventricular valves are shut, so the ventricles are not.
   b. The atria are filling and blood is draining by gravity into the ventricles.
   c. Neither the atria nor the ventricles are filling because the pressure in the heart chambers is too high at this point.
   d. The atria are fully filled already and waiting for the next heartbeat in order to contract and empty into the ventricles.

27. Which of the following describes stroke volume?
   a. The volume of blood ejected by the contracting ventricle.
   b. Heart rate multiplied by end-diastolic volume.
   c. The volume of blood in the ventricle immediately before contraction.
   d. The systolic pressure minus the diastolic pressure.

28. Which of the following is true of blood vessel diameter?
   a. It is regulated by smooth muscle in the tunica adventitia.
   b. It is controlled mainly by sympathetic nerves of the autonomic nervous system.
   c. The smooth muscle of the blood vessel wall is regulated by the cardiovascular centre in the hypothalamus of the brain.
   d. Relaxation of vascular smooth muscle increases peripheral resistance.

29. Where are the baroreceptors controlling blood pressure located?
   a. In the wall of the atria.
   b. In the carotid and aortic sinuses.
   c. In the cardiovascular centre in the medulla oblongata.
   d. In the interventricular septum of the heart.

30. In systemic hypertension, which chamber of the heart is most likely to fail?
   a. Left atrium.
   b. Right atrium.
   c. Left ventricle.
   d. Right ventricle.

31. Which of the following statements regarding parasympathetic stimulation of the heart is correct?
   a. It releases the hormone adrenaline, increasing heart rate.
   b. The heart has no parasympathetic nerve endings, and control of heart activity is under sympathetic control.
   c. It is less important than emotional responses in regulating heart rate.
   d. Parasympathetic supply to the heart is via release of acetylcholine from the vagus nerve.

32. Which of the following increases the risk of ascites?
    a. Liver failure.
    b. Breast tumour with obstructed drainage from axillary lymph nodes.
    c. Hypotension.
    d. Conditions associated with increased plasma protein levels.

33. The pulmonary circulation:
    a. Contains only about 40% of the total circulating blood volume.
    b. Sends oxygenated blood to the lungs via the pulmonary artery.
    c. Is supplied with blood by the left ventricle.
    d. Operates at a much lower blood pressure than the systemic circulation.

34. Which of the following arteries does NOT arise from the aortic arch?
    a. Left subclavian artery.
    b. Right common carotid artery.
    c. Left common carotid artery.
    d. Brachiocephalic artery.

35. Which important vein is formed by the union of the right and left brachiocephalic veins?
    a. Jugular vein.
    b. Carotid vein.
    c. Superior vena cava.
    d. Subclavian vein.

36. The pulse palpable in the wrist is felt from the:
    a. Ulnar artery.
    b. Carpal artery.
    c. Superficial palmar arch.
    d. Radial artery.

37. The circulus arteriosus (circle of Willis):
    a. Is a complete circular channel of arteries lying on the upper surface of the brain.
    b. Provides an important arrangement of anastomotic arteries to ensure constant blood supply to the brain.
    c. Is supplied by arteries including the temporal artery and the internal carotid arteries.
    d. Supplies the cerebral cortex and ventricles, but not the deeper structures of the brain.

38. The superior sagittal sinus drains blood from the superior part of the brain directly into:
    a. The right transverse sinus.
    b. The inferior sagittal sinus.
    c. The straight sinus.
    d. The sagittal sinus.

39. Which of the following is an unpaired artery?
    a. Radial artery.
    b. Internal carotid artery.
    c. Mesenteric artery.
    d. Gastric artery.

40. The cystic vein drains the:
    a. Bladder.
    b. Ovary.
    c. Gall bladder.
    d. Alveoli.

41. The fibular artery is a branch of the:
   a. Popliteal artery.
   b. Femoral artery.
   c. Dorsalis pedis artery.
   d. Posterior tibial artery.

42. Which of the following applies to atherosclerosis but not to arteriosclerosis?
   a. Incidence increases with age.
   b. Fatty deposits form in arterial walls.
   c. There is a strong association with hypertension.
   d. Blood vessel walls become less flexible.

43. The placenta:
   a. Mixes the fetal and maternal blood for transfer of nutrients from mother to baby.
   b. Possesses intervillous spaces that are filled with maternal blood.
   c. Supports the fetus in the final trimester of pregnancy; before that, diffusion across the fetal membranes supplies the growing baby.
   d. Protects the fetus from all infections to which the mother is exposed.

44. In the fetal circulation, the ductus arteriosus:
   a. Shunts blood from the pulmonary artery into the aorta, bypassing the fetal lungs.
   b. Bypasses the fetal liver and delivers blood from the umbilical vein directly into the fetal inferior vena cava.
   c. Shunts blood from the right atrium into the left atrium, bypassing the fetal lungs.
   d. Bypasses the fetal intestines and delivers blood from the umbilical vein directly into the fetal inferior vena cava.

45. The azygos and hemiazygos veins drain which body cavity?
   a. The thoracic cavity.
   b. The cranial cavity.
   c. The abdominal cavity.
   d. The pelvic cavity.

46. Which tissue is present in large amounts in the walls of the aorta but not in, for example, the digital arteries?
   a. Smooth muscle.
   b. Fibrous tissue.
   c. Single-cell thick endothelium.
   d. Elastic tissue.

47. In the healthy, older heart:
   a. The fibrous skeleton softens, giving the heart less support.
   b. The ventricles are usually larger than in the younger heart, compensating for reduced contractility.
   c. The response to adrenaline and noradrenaline is generally more marked, predisposing to heart failure.
   d. It is not possible to improve cardiac function with regular exercise.

48. In Fallot's tetralogy:
   a. The openings to the pulmonary veins are stenosed.
   b. There is usually an atrioseptal defect.
   c. The origin of the aorta is displaced to the left.
   d. Right ventricular hypertrophy is usually evident.

49. Varicose veins are due to:
   a. Aneurysm.
   b. Incompetent valves.
   c. Venous sclerosis.
   d. Venous thrombosis.

50. Which blood vessel links the gastrointestinal tract and the liver?
   a. The hepatic vein.
   b. The hepatic artery.
   c. The hepatic portal vein.
   d. The hepatic mesenteric artery.

CHAPTER 6

The Lymphatic System

Multiple Choice

1. Which of the following is a lymphatic organ?
   a. The heart.
   b. The thymus gland.
   c. The pancreas.
   d. The liver.

2. Peyer's patches are:
   a. Tonsils, found in the throat.
   b. Collections of precursor cells responsible for white blood cell production in the bone marrow.
   c. Important in filtering lymph as it passes through the spleen.
   d. Found in the walls of the small intestine, where they protect against swallowed antigens.

3. Which large lymphatic vessel drains lymph from the intestines?
   a. The thoracic duct.
   b. The right lymphatic duct.
   c. The cisterna chyli.
   d. The subclavian duct.

4. Lymph and plasma:
   a. Are identical in composition.
   b. Are very similar in composition, although plasma contains fewer plasma proteins.
   c. Are very similar in composition, although lymph contains no white blood cells.
   d. Are very similar in composition, although lymph may contain cell debris.

5. Lymph movement along lymphatic vessels is one-way because of:
   a. Rhythmic contraction of smooth muscle in lymphatic vessel walls.
   b. The pumping action of the heart.
   c. Cilia lining lymphatic vessels.
   d. Gravity.

6. The walls of lymph vessels contain:
   a. Skeletal muscle (for the skeletal muscle pump).
   b. The same three layers as veins and arteries.
   c. Elastic tissue in the outer layer.
   d. Endothelium for protection and support.

7. How does the respiratory cycle aid the one-way movement of lymph?
   a. Compression of thoracic structures by the movement of breathing squeezes lymph forward in lymphatic vessels.
   b. Movement of air through the respiratory passageways 'milks' adjacent lymphatic vessels.
   c. Falling pressure in the thorax during inspiration sucks lymph towards the heart.
   d. Increased respiration rate increases blood pressure, which increases the formation and flow of lymph.

8. Lymph nodes:
   a. Filter and clean both blood and lymph.
   b. Are subdivided internally by partitions made of reticular tissue.
   c. Bring lymph in via one afferent lymph vessel.
   d. Are individually enclosed in a fibrous capsule.

9. Which local lymph nodes may be removed as part of the procedure called mastectomy?
   a. Cervical.
   b. Popliteal.
   c. Deep inguinal.
   d. Axillary.

10. The cervical lymph nodes serve the:
    a. Reproductive and other pelvic organs.
    b. Head and neck.
    c. Arm.
    d. Gastrointestinal tract.

11. Macrophages in lymph nodes:
    a. Produce antibodies.
    b. Destroy inorganic particles.
    c. Are phagocytic.
    d. Develop into lymphocytes.

12. Enlargement and inflammation of a lymph node is called:
    a. Lymphadenitis.
    b. Lymphadenopathy.
    c. Lymphangitis.
    d. Lymphoedema.

13. Non-Hodgkin lymphomas:
    a. Are less common than Hodgkin lymphomas.
    b. Usually present with painless lymph node enlargement.
    c. Are malignant tumours of lymphoid tissue.
    d. Never involve the bone marrow.

14. The adenoids are also known as the:
    a. Pharyngeal tonsils.
    b. Palatine tonsils.
    c. Lingual tonsils.
    d. Uvular tonsils.

15. The spleen is located in which abdominal area?
   a. The umbilical region.
   b. The left hypochondriac region.
   c. The right lumbar region.
   d. The left iliac fossa.

16. The spleen:
   a. Lies immediately above the diaphragm.
   b. Stores lymph.
   c. Can store up to 800 mL of blood.
   d. Is an important site of red cell production during fetal development.

17. At which stage in life does thymic atrophy usually begin?
   a. In older age: usually after 70 years.
   b. At puberty.
   c. At birth.
   d. In the fourth decade: somewhere between the ages of 30 and 40.

18. Which defence cell matures within the thymus gland?
   a. T-lymphocytes.
   b. B-lymphocytes.
   c. Natural killer cells.
   d. Plasma cells.

19. Thymosin:
   a. Is produced by the thyroid gland.
   b. Levels usually remain high well into old age.
   c. Stimulates the maturation of lymphatic organs and tissues.
   d. Is released by the reticular tissue of the spleen.

20. Which disorder is strongly associated with thymic enlargement?
   a. Myasthenia gravis.
   b. Hodgkin lymphoma.
   c. Pancreatic cancer.
   d. Duchenne muscular dystrophy.

CHAPTER 7

The Nervous System

Multiple Choice

1. Neurones:
   a. Have many axons.
   b. Have one dendrite.
   c. Are capable of dividing.
   d. Can only synthesise chemical energy (adenosine triphosphate, ATP) from glucose.

2. In nerve cells:
   a. The cell membrane is polarised in the resting state.
   b. Sodium (Na^+) is the principal intracellular cation.
   c. At rest, Na^+ tends to diffuse out of the cells.
   d. Depolarisation occurs when Na^+ floods out of the cells.

3. Nerve impulses:
   a. Can travel either way along a neurone.
   b. Travel more quickly in unmyelinated neurones.
   c. Travel by saltatory conduction in myelinated neurones.
   d. Travel during the refractory period.

4. At the synapse:
   a. The presynaptic neurone has one large synaptic knob.
   b. Neurotransmitters are made just before they are required rather than being stored.
   c. Neurotransmitters diffuse across the synaptic cleft and can only act on specific receptor sites.
   d. Neurotransmitters always have an excitatory effect on the postsynaptic membrane.

5. The fibrous tissue that encloses bundles of nerve fibres is called:
   a. Epineurium.
   b. Endoneurium.
   c. Perineurium.
   d. Myelin.

6. Motor nerves:
   a. Are also known as afferent nerves.
   b. Carry impulses from sensory receptors to the central nervous system.
   c. Include those with endings in the baroreceptors.
   d. Are also known as somatic nerves when they are involved in skeletal muscle contraction (voluntary or reflex).

7. The cells that form and maintain myelin in the central nervous system are:
   a. Oligodendrocytes.
   b. Neurones.
   c. Microglia.
   d. Ependymal cells.

8. The blood-brain barrier is formed by foot processes of:
   a. Oligodendrocytes.
   b. Astrocytes.
   c. Microglia.
   d. Ependymal cells.

9. Which lies outermost in the cranial cavity?
   a. The dura mater.
   b. The arachnoid mater.
   c. The pia mater.
   d. The subarachnoid space.

10. Which fold is formed by the inner layer of dura mater when it sweeps inwards between the cerebral hemispheres?
    a. The falx cerebri.
    b. The falx cerebelli.
    c. The tentorium cerebelli.
    d. None of the above.

11. What is the lower extent of the spinal dura mater?
    a. S3.
    b. S1.
    c. S2.
    d. S4.

12. Diagnostic dyes, local anaesthetics and analgesic drugs are injected into the:
    a. Filum terminale.
    b. Epidural space.
    c. Subdural space.
    d. Subarachnoid space.

13. Which of the meninges extends beyond the spinal cord as the filum terminale?
    a. The dura mater.
    b. The arachnoid mater.
    c. The pia mater.
    d. None of the above.

14. Which of the meninges covers the convolutions of the brain and dips into each fissure?
    a. The dura mater.
    b. The arachnoid mater.
    c. The pia mater.
    d. None of the above.

15. The cerebral aqueduct connects:
    a. The right and left lateral ventricles.
    b. The lateral ventricles and third ventricle.
    c. The third ventricle and fourth ventricle.
    d. The fourth ventricle and spinal cord.

16. Which of the following lies between the cerebellum and the pons?
   a. The lateral ventricles.
   b. The third ventricle.
   c. The fourth ventricle.
   d. None of the above.

17. Cerebrospinal fluid (CSF):
   a. Is secreted at the rate of 5 mL/min.
   b. Is slightly alkaline.
   c. Has a specific gravity of 1.025.
   d. Consists mainly of water, and contains leukocytes, mineral salts, glucose and plasma proteins.

18. An abnormally raised volume of cerebrospinal fluid is known as:
   a. Hydrocephalus.
   b. Cerebral oedema.
   c. Papilloedema.
   d. Herniation.

19. The brain stem includes the:
   a. Cerebrum.
   b. Thalamus.
   c. Pons.
   d. Cerebellum.

20. The amount of blood supplied to the brain is approximately:
   a. 400 mL/min.
   b. 600 mL/min.
   c. 750 mL/min.
   d. 1000 mL/min.

21. The cerebrum:
   a. Is divided by the longitudinal cerebral fissure into anterior and posterior cerebral hemispheres.
   b. Occupies the posterior and middle cranial fossae.
   c. Consists of sulci separated by gyri.
   d. Has a superficial layer that consists of white matter and deeper layers that are composed of grey matter.

22. Which type of fibres connect different parts of the same cerebral hemisphere?
   a. Association fibres.
   b. Commissural fibres.
   c. Projection fibres.
   d. Pyramidal fibres.

23. Which type of tract is the corpus callosum?
   a. An association tract.
   b. A commissural tract.
   c. A projection tract.
   d. A pyramidal tract.

24. The primary motor area of the cerebral cortex:
   a. Lies in the frontal lobe immediately anterior to the central sulcus.
   b. Has areas representing different parts of the body that are proportionally related to their size.
   c. Controls cardiac muscle activity.
   d. Controls voluntary muscle movement on the same side of the body.

25. Where is Broca's area located?
   a. The frontal lobe, immediately anterior to the central sulcus.
   b. The frontal lobe, just superior to the lateral sulcus.
   c. Immediately posterior to the central sulcus.
   d. Posterior to the parieto-occipital sulcus.

26. Wernicke's area is concerned with:
   a. Hearing.
   b. Smell.
   c. Taste.
   d. Speech.

27. The vital centres lie in the:
   a. Midbrain.
   b. Pons.
   c. Medulla oblongata.
   d. Hypothalamus.

28. Brain tumours:
   a. Are nearly always primary tumours.
   b. Usually arise from nerve cells.
   c. Are usually astrocytomas in adults.
   d. Are described as benign when they are slow growing.

29. Coordination and maintenance of posture, balance and equilibrium are the main functions of the:
   a. Reticular formation.
   b. Cerebellum.
   c. Spinal cord.
   d. Cerebral cortex.

30. Intracranial bleeding that most commonly arises from a ruptured berry aneurysm is described as a(n):
   a. Cerebral infarction.
   b. Intracerebral haemorrhage.
   c. Subarachnoid haemorrhage.
   d. Transient ischaemic attack.

31. The microbe that causes shingles is:
   a. Herpes simplex virus.
   b. Varicella-zoster virus.
   c. *Neisseria meningitidis.*
   d. *Streptococcus pneumoniae.*

32. The type of dementia that is inherited as an autosomal dominant disorder is:
   a. Creutzfeldt-Jakob's disease.
   b. Parkinson's disease.
   c. Alzheimer's disease.
   d. Huntington's disease.

33. The spinal cord:
   a. Has an anterior shallow median fissure and a posterior deep posterior median septum.
   b. Has white matter in the centre, surrounded by grey matter.
   c. Is about 90 cm long in adult males.
   d. Contains white matter arranged in the shape of the letter H.

34. Which sensory nerve pathways do NOT decussate in the spinal cord?
   a. Pain.
   b. Temperature.
   c. Touch.
   d. Proprioception.

35. The cell bodies of lower motor neurones are located in the:
   a. Cerebrum.
   b. Anterior horn of grey matter of spinal cord.
   c. Posterior horn of grey matter in spinal cord.
   d. Lateral column of white matter in spinal cord.

36. Multiple sclerosis is classified as:
   a. A demyelinating disease.
   b. A lower motor neurone disease.
   c. An upper motor neurone disease.
   d. Compression of the spinal cord.

37. When bright light reaches the eye, the pupil constricts. This is an example of:
   a. A spinal reflex.
   b. A stretch reflex.
   c. An autonomic reflex.
   d. A voluntary movement.

38. The smallest plexus is the:
   a. Coccygeal.
   b. Cervical.
   c. Sacral.
   d. Brachial.

39. The phrenic nerve originates from:
   a. Cervical nerve roots 1, 2, 3 and 4.
   b. Cervical nerve roots 3, 4 and 5.
   c. The lower four cervical and 1st thoracic nerve roots.
   d. The first three and part of 4th lumbar nerve roots.

40. Which is the largest branch of the brachial plexus?
   a. The axillary nerve.
   b. The musculocutaneous nerve.
   c. The iliohypogastric nerve.
   d. The radial nerve.

41. The largest nerve in the body is the:
a. Great auricular nerve.
b. Radial nerve.
c. Femoral nerve.
d. Sciatic nerve.

42. The external anal sphincter is supplied by the:
a. Tibial nerve.
b. Common peroneal nerve.
c. Pudendal nerve.
d. Coccygeal plexus.

43. The cranial nerve with the most extensive distribution to internal organs is the:
a. Vagus nerve.
b. Accessory nerve.
c. Trochlear nerve.
d. Abducent nerve.

44. Which of the following is NOT a branch of the trigeminal nerve?
a. Trochlear nerve.
b. Ophthalmic nerve.
c. Maxillary nerve.
d. Mandibular nerve.

45. The cranial nerve essential for the swallowing and gag reflexes is the:
a. Glossopharyngeal nerve.
b. Hypoglossal nerve.
c. Accessory nerve.
d. Vagus nerve.

46. Which of the following are NOT mixed nerves?
a. The facial nerves.
b. The vestibulocochlear nerves.
c. The glossopharyngeal nerves.
d. The vagus nerves.

47. The sympathetic nervous system:
a. Is a craniosacral outflow.
b. Has five prevertebral ganglia in the abdominal cavity.
c. Does not have postsynaptic neurones to the heart.
d. Sometimes has sympathetic cholinergic nerves as its postsynaptic neurones.

48. The parasympathetic nervous system:
a. Has a chain of ganglia on each side of the spinal cord.
b. Always uses acetylcholine as the neurotransmitter at both pre- and postganglionic synapses.
c. Innervates the adrenal medulla releasing noradrenaline when stimulated.
d. Has long postsynaptic neurones.

49. Which of the following is NOT an effect of sympathetic stimulation?
a. Fight or flight response.
b. Greatly increased metabolic rate.
c. Increased motility and secretion in stomach and small intestine.
d. Goose flesh.

50. If referred pain is present in the loin and groin, the tissue of origin would be the:
a. Heart.
b. Uterus.
c. Appendix.
d. Kidney and ureter.

CHAPTER 8

The Special Senses

Multiple Choice

1. The external acoustic meatus:
   a. Is J-shaped and about 5 cm long.
   b. Carries sound waves to the inner ear.
   c. Is lined with skin containing ceruminous glands.
   d. Is normally closed but when there is unequal pressure across it, e.g., at high altitude, it can be opened by swallowing or yawning, and the ears 'pop', equalising the pressure again.

2. The tympanic cavity:
   a. Is filled with serous fluid.
   b. Contains the utricle.
   c. Is largely bounded by the temporal bone.
   d. Is lined with squamous epithelium.

3. Which of the auditory ossicles is anvil-shaped and has long and short processes?
   a. The malleus.
   b. The incus.
   c. The stapes.
   d. The saccule.

4. Which is NOT part of the inner ear?
   a. The vestibule.
   b. The semicircular canals.
   c. The cochlea.
   d. The pharyngotympanic tube.

5. In the inner ear:
   a. The membranous labyrinth lies within the bony labyrinth.
   b. The bony labyrinth is filled with endolymph.
   c. The auditory receptors are dendrites of specialised efferent nerve endings.
   d. The cochlear duct contains perilymph.

6. Sound is perceived by the:
   a. Inner ear.
   b. Cochlear hair cells.
   c. Auditory ossicles.
   d. Temporal lobe of the cerebrum.

7. Conductive hearing loss can be caused by:
   a. Ototoxic drugs, e.g., aminoglycoside antibiotics.
   b. Acute otitis media.
   c. Long-term exposure to excessive noise.
   d. Ménière's disease.

8. Hair cells for balance are located in:
   a. The utricle.
   b. The semicircular canals.
   c. The spiral organ.
   d. The basilar membrane.

9. Which is the middle layer of the eyeball wall?
   a. The sclera.
   b. The cornea.
   c. The uveal tract.
   d. The retina.

10. The choroid:
    a. Lines the posterior five-sixths of the sclera.
    b. Is devoid of blood vessels.
    c. Gives attachment to the extrinsic muscles of the eye.
    d. Gives attachment to the intrinsic muscles of the eye.

11. Which of the following is NOT true of the ciliary body?
    a. It gives attachment to the lens through suspensory ligaments.
    b. The ciliary muscle consists of radiating muscle fibres that dilate the pupil when stimulated.
    c. It contains epithelial cells that secrete aqueous fluid.
    d. It is supplied by parasympathetic branches of the third cranial nerve.

12. Eye colour is determined by the:
    a. Cornea.
    b. Choroid.
    c. Iris.
    d. Retina.

13. Opacity of the lens is caused by:
    a. Retinal detachment.
    b. Colour blindness.
    c. Strabismus.
    d. Cataracts.

14. The fovea centralis is found in the:
    a. Macula lutea.
    b. Optic disc.
    c. Ciliary body.
    d. Iris.

15. The central retinal artery and vein are encased within the optic nerve that enters the eye at the:
    a. Macula lutea.
    b. Optic disc.
    c. Fovea centralis.
    d. Scleral venous sinus.

16. Structures in the eye that have no blood supply include:
   a. The cornea.
   b. The lens.
   c. The lens capsule.
   d. All of the above.

17. Normal intraocular pressure is approximately
   a. 2–8 mmHg.
   b. 10–20 mmHg.
   c. 20–40 mmHg.
   d. None of the above.

18. Raised intraocular pressure causes:
   a. Retinal detachment.
   b. Strabismus.
   c. Cataracts.
   d. Glaucoma.

19. The optic tracts contain:
   a. Nasal fibres from one eye and temporal fibres from the other eye.
   b. Nasal and temporal fibres from the same eye.
   c. Nerve fibres from the visual area in the cerebrum.
   d. Nerve fibres from the visual area in the cerebellum.

20. Where do the optic radiations terminate?
   a. The lateral geniculate bodies.
   b. The occipital lobes of cerebrum.
   c. The cerebellum.
   d. The optic chiasma.

21. Which of the following is involved in producing a clear visual image of nearby objects?
   a. Refraction of light rays.
   b. A change in the size of the pupils.
   c. Accommodation of the lens.
   d. All of the above.

22. Which of the following have the longest wavelength?
   a. Microwaves.
   b. Violet light rays.
   c. X-rays.
   d. Gamma rays.

23. Which of the following are sensitive to colour?
   a. Rods.
   b. Cones.
   c. Rhodopsin.
   d. All of the above.

24. The ability to judge the speed and distance of an approaching vehicle is impaired in:
   a. Colour blindness.
   b. Dark adaptation.
   c. Binocular vision.
   d. Monocular vision.

25. The abducent nerve supplies the:
   a. Medial rectus muscles.
   b. Superior oblique muscles.
   c. Lateral rectus muscles.
   d. Intrinsic muscles of the iris and ciliary body.

26. Which of the extraocular muscles rotates the eyeball upwards and outwards?
   a. The superior rectus.
   b. The inferior rectus.
   c. The superior oblique.
   d. The inferior oblique.

27. The tarsal glands are found in the:
   a. Eyebrows.
   b. Eyelids.
   c. Lacrimal apparatus.
   d. Conjunctiva.

28. The sense of taste is carried by all of the following, EXCEPT:
   a. Glossopharyngeal nerve.
   b. Facial nerve.
   c. Vagus nerve.
   d. Olfactory nerve.

29. What is the final destination of impulses travelling along the sensory taste fibres?
   a. The parietal lobe of the cerebral cortex.
   b. The frontal lobe of the cerebral cortex.
   c. The temporal lobe of the cerebral cortex.
   d. The occipital lobe of the cerebral cortex.

30. By the age of 40 years, most adults require spectacles for reading due to development of:
   a. Cataracts.
   b. Presbyopia.
   c. Presbycusis.
   d. Otosclerosis.

CHAPTER 9

The Endocrine System

Multiple Choice

1. Glands with secondary endocrine functions include the:
a. Thymus.
b. Pineal.
c. Pituitary.
d. Parathyroids.

2. Which is a peptide hormone?
a. Cortisone.
b. Thyroxine.
c. Insulin.
d. Aldosterone.

3. Secretion of which hormone is regulated by a positive feedback mechanism?
a. Luteinising hormone (LH).
b. Thyroxine.
c. Oxytocin.
d. Glucagon.

4. What is the average weight of the pituitary gland?
a. 250 mg.
b. 500 mg.
c. 25 g.
d. 50 g.

5. The internal carotid artery supplies the:
a. Thyroid gland.
b. Pituitary gland.
c. Pineal gland.
d. Thymus gland.

6. Pituicytes are found in the:
a. Anterior lobe of the pituitary.
b. Posterior lobe of the pituitary.
c. Anterior and posterior lobes of the pituitary.
d. Intermediate lobe of the pituitary.

7. Which of the following statements regarding the pituitary gland is true?
a. The pituitary portal system carries blood from the hypothalamus to the posterior lobe.
b. Releasing hormones are produced by the anterior lobe.
c. Trophic hormones are produced by the posterior lobe.
d. Oxytocin is released by axon terminals in the posterior lobe.

8. Acromegaly:
   a. Occurs in children.
   b. Is associated with hypersecretion of adrenocorticotrophic hormone (ACTH).
   c. Causes excessive growth of the hands and feet.
   d. Is a tumour of the posterior pituitary.

9. The most abundant hormone synthesised by the anterior pituitary is:
   a. Growth hormone (GH).
   b. Thyroid stimulating hormone (TSH).
   c. ACTH.
   d. Prolactin.

10. Which hormone is associated with the sleep pattern and jet lag?
   a. GH.
   b. Thyroid hormone.
   c. Prolactin.
   d. ACTH.

11. Levels of which hormone fall during the night?
   a. GH.
   b. TSH.
   c. ACTH.
   d. Antidiuretic hormone (ADH).

12. Which of the following is a sex hormone?
   a. LH.
   b. Follicle stimulating hormone (FSH).
   c. Both LH and FSH.
   d. Neither LH nor FSH.

13. Oxytocin:
   a. Causes contraction of uterine muscle during childbirth.
   b. Stimulates contraction of milk ducts and ejection of milk.
   c. Levels rise during sexual arousal.
   d. All of the above.

14. After drinking a large volume of fluid, the blood level of ADH will:
   a. Increase.
   b. Decrease.
   c. Decrease and then increase shortly afterwards.
   d. Remain unchanged.

15. Which is NOT a target tissue for ADH?
   a. The distal convoluted tubules of the kidney.
   b. The proximal convoluted tubules of the kidney.
   c. The collecting ducts of the kidney.
   d. Smooth muscle in the walls of small arteries.

16. The approximate weight of the thyroid gland is:
   a. 25 g.
   b. 50 g.
   c. 100 g.
   d. 150 g.

17. Tetany is associated with:
a. Hypothyroidism.
b. Hyperthyroidism.
c. Hypoparathyroidism.
d. Hyperparathyroidism

18. Secretion of T3 and T4 begins in which month of fetal life?
a. Third month.
b. Fourth month.
c. Fifth month.
d. Sixth month.

19. Effects of hypothyroidism include:
a. Weight gain.
b. Anxiety.
c. Hair loss.
d. Heat intolerance.

20. Simple goitre is associated with:
a. Bulging eyes (exophthalmos).
b. Signs of hyperthyroidism.
c. Enlargement of the thyroid gland.
d. All of the above.

21. The hormone calcitonin:
a. Is secreted by the follicular cells of the thyroid gland.
b. Promotes storage of calcium in the bones.
c. Raises lowered blood calcium levels.
d. Increases reabsorption of calcium by the renal tubules.

22. Which of the following is a glucocorticoid hormone?
a. Aldosterone.
b. Corticosterone.
c. Testosterone.
d. All of the above.

23. Glucocorticoid hormones do NOT:
a. Increase plasma glucose levels.
b. Increase free fatty acid levels in the plasma.
c. Increase plasma calcium levels.
d. Increase plasma levels of amino acids.

24. Which of the following organs/tissues is NOT involved in activation of the renin-angiotensin-aldosterone system?
a. Kidney.
b. Liver.
c. Lung.
d. Heart.

25. Features of the fight or flight response include:
a. Increased blood pressure.
b. Decreased metabolic rate.
c. Constriction of the pupils.
d. All of the above.

26. Insulin is secreted by:
   a. Alpha cells of the pancreatic islets.
   b. Beta cells of the pancreatic islets.
   c. Delta cells of the pancreatic islets.
   d. Sympathetic nerve endings in the adrenal medulla.

27. Insulin:
   a. Is a polypeptide hormone consisting of about 25 amino acids.
   b. Increases glycogenolysis.
   c. Increases uptake of glucose into cells.
   d. Secretion is stimulated by cortisol.

28. Type 2 diabetes mellitus:
   a. Is also known as diabetes insipidus.
   b. Usually affects children.
   c. Always requires treatment with insulin injections.
   d. Will already have caused long-term complications in 25% of patients at the time of diagnosis.

29. Leptin is secreted by:
   a. Adipose tissue.
   b. The placenta.
   c. The pineal gland.
   d. The gastric mucosa.

30. Which locally acting hormone is released from mast cells in the allergic response?
   a. Serotonin.
   b. Prostaglandins.
   c. Histamine.
   d. Thromboxanes.

CHAPTER 10

The Respiratory System

Multiple Choice

1. Which of the following contributes to the formation of the nasal septum?
a. The vomer.
b. The sphenoid bone.
c. The hard palate.
d. The nasal bone.

2. How many pairs of nares (nostrils) are found in the upper respiratory tract?
a. One.
b. Two.
c. Three.
d. Four.

3. The nasal conchae:
a. Are folds of the nasal bone.
b. Help to lighten the skull.
c. Contain defence cells that intercept inhaled antigens.
d. Increase the internal surface area of the nasal cavity.

4. The pharynx extends from the base of the skull to the level of which of the cervical vertebrae?
a. Fourth.
b. Fifth.
c. Sixth.
d. Seventh.

5. The two tiny openings in the laryngopharynx communicate with:
a. The oropharynx.
b. The maxillary sinus.
c. The middle ear.
d. The ethmoid sinus.

6. This cartilage, which is part of the larynx, is broader at the back than at the front and encircles the laryngeal opening. It is the:
a. Epiglottis.
b. Cricoid cartilage.
c. Arytenoid cartilage.
d. Thyroid cartilage.

7. Rhinoviruses are frequent causes of:
   a. The common cold.
   b. Influenza.
   c. Allergic rhinitis.
   d. Diphtheria.

8. When the muscles controlling the vocal cords are relaxed:
   a. The glottis is closed.
   b. There is free air flow through the larynx.
   c. The voice becomes high pitched.
   d. The vocal cords are said to be adducted.

9. What is the carina?
   a. The area of the lung where the primary bronchi enter.
   b. The most inferior part of the trachea.
   c. The largest of the tracheal cartilages.
   d. The space between the vocal cords.

10. Which of the following describes the relationship between the trachea and the oesophagus?
   a. The oesophagus is anterior to the trachea.
   b. The posterior wall of the trachea lies against the oesophagus.
   c. The oesophageal wall contains the trachealis muscle, which facilitates swallowing.
   d. The openings of the C-shaped tracheal cartilages lie immediately behind the oesophagus.

11. Which of the following is associated with the cough reflex?
   a. Irritation of the upper respiratory tract stimulates vagal input to the respiratory centre.
   b. The glottis must be completely open in order to increase pressure in the lungs.
   c. Relaxation of the abdominal muscles allows the diaphragm to contract fully.
   d. Immediately prior to the cough action, there must be a full breath out.

12. The medial surface of the lung:
   a. Lies against the ribcage.
   b. Is covered by the parietal pleura.
   c. Faces the heart.
   d. Is grooved to accommodate the intercostal muscles.

13. Which of the following is NOT found at the hilum of the lung?
   a. Two pulmonary arteries.
   b. Two pulmonary veins.
   c. The primary bronchus.
   d. Nerves supplying the lung.

14. Which of the following is NOT in direct contact with the parietal pleura?
   a. The heart.
   b. The ribcage.
   c. The diaphragm.
   d. The lung.

15. The lung substance is rich in:
   a. Supportive fibrous tissue.
   b. Elastic connective tissue.
   c. Cartilage, for support.
   d. Adipose tissue, for energy.

16. The respiratory membrane:
a. Lines the upper respiratory tract.
b. Covers the lung surface.
c. Includes the alveolar wall.
d. Adheres to the inside of the ribcage.

17. The lungs are not symmetrical. Which of the following applies to the right lung but not to the left?
a. The right lung possesses two lobes.
b. The right lung sits higher in the chest than the left lung.
c. The right lung is smaller than the left lung because the heart is not central.
d. The base of the right lung lies immediately above the diaphragm.

18. Atopic asthma:
a. Usually arises in adulthood.
b. Is not associated with allergy.
c. Frequently runs in families.
d. Is associated with excessive dilation of the airways.

19. What is the function of septal cells in the alveolar wall?
a. Phagocytosis of bacteria and other foreign materials.
b. Regulation of air flow.
c. Production of pleural fluid.
d. Secretion of surfactant.

20. Collapse of all or part of the lung is called:
a. Pneumothorax.
b. Atelectasis.
c. Emphysema.
d. Pleurisy.

21. Surfactant:
a. Reduces surface tension in the alveoli.
b. Lubricates the visceral and parietal pleura.
c. Facilitates gas exchange across the alveolar wall.
d. Has antibacterial properties and protects against infection.

22. External respiration:
a. Is the physical action of breathing.
b. Refers to gas exchange in the lungs.
c. Means the excretion of carbon dioxide during exhalation.
d. Refers to diffusion of oxygen from the bloodstream into the tissues.

23. Which of the following is true?
a. There are 11 pairs of ribs and 11 pairs of intercostal muscles.
b. There are 12 pairs of ribs and 11 pairs of intercostal muscles.
c. There are 11 pairs of ribs and 12 pairs of intercostal muscles.
d. There are 12 pairs of ribs and 12 pairs of intercostal muscles.

24. Which of the following is/are classed as accessory muscle(s) of respiration?
a. The diaphragm.
b. The external intercostals.
c. The deltoid.
d. The internal intercostals.

25. Which of the following is true of the diaphragm?
a. It contracts in response to stimulation by the vagus nerve.
b. Its central tendon is perforated by the aorta.
c. It is a dome-shaped muscle forming the floor of the abdominal cavity.
d. When its fibres contract, the diaphragm rises into the thorax.

26. The intrapleural space:
a. Lies between the pleura and the lung surface.
b. Contains about 200 mL of pleural fluid.
c. Is kept at subatmospheric pressure.
d. Is occupied by the heart, great vessels and other important structures.

27. Which of the following can be used to calculate the residual volume of the lungs?
a. Tidal volume subtracted from vital capacity.
b. Inspiratory reserve volume and expiratory reserve volume subtracted from total lung capacity.
c. Inspiratory reserve volume subtracted from inspiratory capacity.
d. Vital capacity subtracted from total lung capacity.

28. Which gas comprises 78% of atmospheric air?
a. Nitrogen.
b. Oxygen.
c. Carbon dioxide.
d. Hydrogen.

29. The partial pressure of oxygen (PO_2) of blood leaving the lungs in the pulmonary vein is:
a. 5.4 kPa.
b. 9.1 kPa.
c. 13.3 kPa.
d. 16.8 kPa.

30. The PO_2 of blood arriving at the lungs in the pulmonary artery:
a. Is the same as the PO_2 of blood in the pulmonary vein.
b. Is higher than the PO_2 of blood in the aorta.
c. Is the same as the PO_2 of blood leaving the tissues.
d. Is less than the PO_2 of blood in the vena cava.

31. What proportion of blood oxygen is carried dissolved in plasma?
a. 50%.
b. 1.5%.
c. 15%.
d. 20%.

32. What is the role of neurones in the pneumotaxic area in the control of breathing?
a. They set the basic rhythm of breathing.
b. They trigger forced expiration.
c. They detect the degree of stretch in the lung tissue.
d. They increase the rate and/or depth of breathing when required.

33. Peripheral chemoreceptors in the carotid arteries and aorta increase respiratory effort when stimulated by:
a. Rising blood pressure.
b. Increased blood oxygen levels.
c. Decreased blood pH.
d. Reduced blood H^+ concentration.

CHAPTER 11

Introduction to Nutrition

Multiple Choice

1. Nutrients do not include:
a. Carbohydrates.
b. Proteins.
c. Non-starch polysaccharides.
d. Mineral salts and trace elements.

2. If body mass index (BMI) is 22.5, an individual will be:
a. Underweight.
b. Within the normal range.
c. Overweight.
d. Obese.

3. If BMI is 25.2, an individual will be:
a. Underweight.
b. Within the normal range.
c. Overweight.
d. Obese.

4. The most concentrated form of energy comes from:
a. Fats.
b. Non-starch polysaccharides.
c. Proteins.
d. Carbohydrates.

5. Which foodstuff is not considered to be one of the fruit and vegetable food group?
a. Apples.
b. Pure fruit smoothies.
c. Sweet potatoes.
d. Salad.

6. Amino acids are a constituent of:
a. Carbohydrates.
b. Proteins.
c. Non-starch polysaccharides.
d. Mineral salts and trace elements.

7. Saturated fats:
   a. Are also known as triglycerides.
   b. Usually come from plants.
   c. Are liquids at room temperature.
   d. Consist of carbon, hydrogen and oxygen, the hydrogen and oxygen being in the same proportions as water.

8. Which is an oily fish?
   a. Haddock.
   b. Cod.
   c. Snapper.
   d. Salmon.

9. Fat-soluble vitamins include:
   a. A.
   b. B.
   c. C.
   d. All of the above.

10. Which mineral is NOT essential for muscular contraction?
   a. Iodine.
   b. Sodium.
   c. Potassium.
   d. Calcium.

11. The recommended daily fluid intake for adults is:
   a. 0.5–1 L.
   b. 1–1.5 L.
   c. 1.5–2 L.
   d. 2–2.5 L.

12. High-density lipoprotein:
   a. Carries cholesterol from body cells to the liver.
   b. Is harmful to health when blood levels are excessive.
   c. Is synthesised from arachidonic acid.
   d. Cannot be synthesised by the body, so is an essential nutrient.

13. Menstruating women require more of which substance than their non-menstruating counterparts?
   a. Energy.
   b. Protein.
   c. Calcium.
   d. Iron.

14. Deficiency of which mineral predisposes to goitre?
   a. Potassium.
   b. Iodine.
   c. Sodium.
   d. Phosphate.

15. Deficiency of which substance predisposes to megaloblastic anaemia?
  a. Calcium.
  b. Iron.
  c. Vitamin K.
  d. Vitamin B_{12}.

16. Vitamin C:
  a. Deficiency becomes apparent after 1–2 months.
  b. Is also known as niacin.
  c. Is a fat-soluble vitamin.
  d. Is easily destroyed by heat and salting.

17. Daily supplements for all adults over 65 are recommended for:
  a. Vitamin A.
  b. Vitamin B.
  c. Vitamin C.
  d. Vitamin D.

18. An example of malabsorption specific to one nutrient only is:
  a. Cystic fibrosis.
  b. Pernicious anaemia.
  c. Tropical sprue.
  d. Kwashiorkor.

19. In marasmus:
  a. Growth in children is retarded.
  b. There is associated oedema.
  c. There is often a history of infection, e.g., measles.
  d. Liver damage is common.

20. Which is NOT true about leptin?
  a. It is released from adipose tissue.
  b. It is involved in puberty.
  c. It is involved in lactation.
  d. Its release suppresses the appetite.

CHAPTER 12

The Digestive System

Multiple Choice

1. The physiological term for eating and drinking is:
   a. Ingestion.
   b. Propulsion.
   c. Absorption.
   d. Digestion.

2. The layers forming the walls of the alimentary tract include:
   a. The mucosa.
   b. The submucosa.
   c. The serosa.
   d. All of the above.

3. The accessory organs of digestion do NOT include the:
   a. Salivary glands.
   b. Pancreas.
   c. Duodenum.
   d. Liver.

4. The serous membrane that lines the abdominal wall is the:
   a. Visceral peritoneum.
   b. Parietal peritoneum.
   c. Mesentery.
   d. Greater omentum.

5. Which organ is retroperitoneal?
   a. Liver.
   b. Stomach.
   c. Kidney.
   d. Small intestine.

6. In the alimentary tract, the muscle layer:
   a. Is arranged with the circular fibres outside the longitudinal fibres.
   b. Has its plexus outermost.
   c. Produces peristalsis through contraction and relaxation of the longitudinal muscle fibres.
   d. Has thickened rings of circular muscle known as sphincters.

7. The myenteric plexus is located in the:
   a. Mucosa.
   b. Submucosa.
   c. Muscle layer.
   d. Serosa.

8. What are the effects of parasympathetic stimulation on the alimentary tract?
   a. Increased muscular activity.
   b. Increased glandular secretion.
   c. Both a. and b.
   d. Neither a. nor b.

9. Goblet cells secrete:
   a. Mucus.
   b. Saliva.
   c. Amylase.
   d. Bile.

10. Which of the following is NOT a boundary of the oral cavity?
    a. The lips.
    b. The palate.
    c. The tongue.
    d. The oesophagus.

11. Which nerve supplies the voluntary tongue muscles?
    a. The hypoglossal nerve.
    b. The mandibular nerve.
    c. The facial nerve.
    d. The glossopharyngeal nerve.

12. The sensory receptors for taste are present in:
    a. The soft palate.
    b. The pharynx.
    c. The epiglottis.
    d. All of the above.

13. All the deciduous teeth should be visible by the age of:
    a. 6 months.
    b. 24 months.
    c. 6 years.
    d. 21 years.

14. What secures a tooth in its socket?
    a. The pulp cavity.
    b. The dentine.
    c. The enamel.
    d. The cementum.

15. The ducts of which salivary glands open into the mouth beside the second upper molar tooth?
    a. The parotid glands.
    b. The submandibular glands.
    c. The sublingual glands.
    d. The adrenal glands.

16. The facial artery supplies the:
    a. Tongue.
    b. Teeth.
    c. Pharynx.
    d. Oesophagus.

17. The oesophagus passes through the diaphragm at the level of which vertebra?
    a. T8.
    b. T10.
    c. T11.
    d. T12.

18. Dysphagia is:
    a. Difficulty swallowing.
    b. Vomiting blood.
    c. Passing blood in the faeces.
    d. Feeling of sickness.

19. Which anatomical feature(s) minimises gastric reflux?
    a. The attachment of the stomach to the diaphragm.
    b. The acute angle at the junction of the oesophagus and the diaphragm.
    c. Increased tone of the lower oesophageal sphincter during increased intra-abdominal pressure.
    d. All of the above.

20. Which organ has three layers of muscle fibres?
    a. The oesophagus.
    b. The stomach.
    c. The small intestine.
    d. The large intestine.

21. Pepsinogen is secreted by:
    a. Mucous neck cells.
    b. Parietal cells.
    c. Chief cells.
    d. All of the above.

22. The condition where part of the stomach protrudes though the oesophageal opening in the diaphragm is known as a(n):
    a. Hiatus hernia.
    b. Inguinal hernia.
    c. Umbilical hernia.
    d. Peritoneal hernia.

23. Secretin is released in which phase(s) of gastric secretion?
    a. The cephalic phase.
    b. The gastric phase.
    c. The intestinal phase.
    d. All of the above.

24. A meal high in which of the following remains longest in the stomach?
    a. Carbohydrate.
    b. Protein.
    c. Fat.
    d. Fibre.

25. Vomiting:
   a. Is a voluntary process.
   b. Is accompanied by strong reverse waves of gastric peristalsis.
   c. Can lead to serious acidosis.
   d. Is coordinated by the cerebrum.

26. Which is the longest?
   a. The large intestine.
   b. The duodenum.
   c. The jejunum.
   d. The ileum.

27. In ulcerative colitis:
   a. There is a high risk of malignancy developing.
   b. Any part of the digestive tract can be affected and the terminal ileum is typically involved.
   c. The entire thickness of the intestinal wall is affected.
   d. Ulcers and fistulae are common.

28. The hepatopancreatic sphincter is located in the:
   a. Stomach.
   b. Duodenum.
   c. Jejunum.
   d. Ileum.

29. Aggregated lymph follicles (Peyer's patches) are found in the:
   a. Duodenum.
   b. Jejunum.
   c. Ileum.
   d. Large intestine.

30. How many days does replacement of the entire epithelium of the small intestine take?
   a. 2–3 days.
   b. 3–5 days.
   c. 5–8 days.
   d. 8–12 days.

31. Which condition predisposes to malignancy in the alimentary tract?
   a. Tropical sprue.
   b. Coeliac disease.
   c. Diverticular disease.
   d. Barrett's oesophagus.

32. Which is a constituent of pancreatic juice?
   a. Trypsinogen.
   b. Cholecystokinin.
   c. Pepsinogen.
   d. Intrinsic factor.

33. Hepatitis B:
   a. Is spread by the faecal-oral route.
   b. Has a carrier state.
   c. Has an incubation period of 5 to 18 days.
   d. Is a mild illness.

34. Which vitamin is absorbed into the lacteals?
  a. B.
  b. C.
  c. D.
  d. Folic acid.

35. Vitamin B_{12} is absorbed in the:
  a. Stomach.
  b. Duodenum.
  c. Terminal ileum.
  d. Large intestine.

36. Which part of the large intestine has an S-shaped curve?
  a. The caecum.
  b. The sigmoid colon.
  c. The rectum.
  d. The anal canal.

37. In adults, the approximate length of the anal canal is:
  a. 6.2 cm.
  b. 5.8 cm.
  c. 4.8 cm.
  d. 3.8 cm.

38. The arterial supply to the caecum is via the:
  a. Superior mesenteric artery.
  b. Inferior mesenteric artery.
  c. Middle rectal artery.
  d. Inferior rectal artery.

39. Which is the largest gland?
  a. The pancreas.
  b. The liver.
  c. The parotids.
  d. The adrenals.

40. Which is the largest lobe of the liver?
  a. Right.
  b. Left.
  c. Caudate.
  d. Quadrate.

41. How is the liver related to the diaphragm anatomically?
  a. Anteriorly.
  b. Posteriorly.
  c. Laterally.
  d. All of the above.

42. Which of the following are bile acids?
  a. Cholic acid.
  b. Chenodeoxycholic acid.
  c. Both of the above.
  d. Neither of the above.

43. Uric acid is a breakdown product of:
    a. Linoleic acid.
    b. Deoxyribonucleic acid.
    c. Amino acids.
    d. Creatinine.

44. Intrahepatic jaundice can be caused by:
    a. Viral hepatitis.
    b. Impacted gallstones.
    c. Excessive haemolysis.
    d. A tumour of the head of the pancreas.

45. In the biliary tract:
    a. The right and left hepatic ducts join just before passing out of the portal fissure.
    b. The hepatic duct is joined by the cystic duct from the liver.
    c. The right and left hepatic ducts merge forming the common bile duct.
    d. The common bile duct joins the pancreatic duct at the hepatopancreatic ampulla.

46. A gallstone lodged in the biliary tract will cause jaundice if it is impacted in the:
    a. Gall bladder.
    b. Cystic duct.
    c. Common bile duct.
    d. All of the above.

47. What is/are the function(s) of the gall bladder?
    a. A reservoir for bile.
    b. Concentration of bile.
    c. Release of stored bile.
    d. All of the above.

48. Metabolic rate:
    a. Is higher in women than men.
    b. Increases with age.
    c. Increases during starvation.
    d. Increases during a fever.

49. Which is NOT a central metabolic pathway?
    a. The citric acid cycle.
    b. Glycolysis.
    c. Deamination.
    d. Oxidative phosphorylation.

50. An example of an anaerobic metabolic pathway is:
    a. The citric acid cycle.
    b. Glycolysis.
    c. Deamination.
    d. Oxidative phosphorylation.

CHAPTER 13

The Urinary System

Multiple Choice

1. Which structure lies anteriorly to the left kidney?
a. The liver.
b. The duodenum.
c. The colon.
d. The pancreas.

2. The concave medial border of the kidney is called the:
a. Capsule.
b. Cortex.
c. Medulla.
d. Hilum.

3. The funnel-shaped structure that collects urine formed by the kidney is the:
a. Hilum.
b. Renal papilla.
c. Renal pelvis.
d. Ureter.

4. The functional unit of the kidney is the:
a. Nephron.
b. Collecting duct.
c. Glomerulus.
d. Medullary loop (of Henle).

5. What percentage of the cardiac output do the kidneys receive?
a. 10%.
b. 20%.
c. 30%.
d. 40%.

6. The afferent arteriole in the nephron:
a. Subdivides into a cluster of tiny arterial capillaries, forming the glomerulus.
b. Is the blood vessel leading away from the glomerulus.
c. Is smaller in diameter than the efferent arteriole.
d. Divides into a second peritubular capillary network, which wraps around the remainder of the tubule.

7. Which of the following is (are) involved in the formation of urine?
   a. Filtration.
   b. Selective reabsorption.
   c. Secretion.
   d. All of the above.

8. Which of the following is NOT a normal constituent of glomerular filtrate?
   a. Water.
   b. Glucose.
   c. Creatinine.
   d. Plasma proteins.

9. What is the glomerular filtration rate (GFR) in normal healthy adults?
   a. 90 mL/min.
   b. 125 mL/min.
   c. 160 mL/min.
   d. 200 mL/min.

10. Which of the following hormones does NOT influence selective reabsorption of water?
    a. Parathyroid hormone.
    b. Antidiuretic hormone.
    c. Aldosterone.
    d. Atrial natriuretic peptide.

11. The characteristics of urine include:
    a. Specific gravity between 1005 and 1010.
    b. pH around 6.
    c. Volume 750–1000 mL per day in adults.
    d. Water 80%.

12. pH balance of the blood is maintained by processes that occur in the:
    a. Glomerulus.
    b. Proximal convoluted tubule.
    c. Medullary loop (of Henle).
    d. Distal convoluted tubule.

13. The most common cation (positively charged ion) in extracellular fluid is:
    a. Sodium.
    b. Potassium.
    c. Calcium.
    d. Urea.

14. In which condition(s) is the amount of sodium excreted in the urine increased?
    a. Pyrexia.
    b. High environmental temperature.
    c. During sustained physical exercise.
    d. All of the above.

15. Where is the plasma protein angiotensinogen produced?
    a. The lungs.
    b. The liver.
    c. The proximal convoluted tubules of the nephrons.
    d. The adrenal cortex.

16. When chronic kidney disease is accompanied by deficiency of the hormone erythropoietin, this will lead to:
  a. Acidosis.
  b. Anaemia.
  c. Hypertension.
  d. Polyuria.

17. The total capacity of the bladder in adults is about:
  a. 100 mL.
  b. 400 mL.
  c. 600 mL.
  d. 1000 mL.

18. How much urine does the urinary bladder contain when the individual becomes aware of the need to pass urine?
  a. 200–300 mL.
  b. 300–400 mL.
  c. 400–500 mL.
  d. 500–600 mL.

19. Dysuria is:
  a. Passing large volumes of urine.
  b. Passing urine during the night.
  c. Urine output less than 400 mL/day.
  d. Pain on passing urine.

20. Cystitis is:
  a. Associated with frequency of micturition.
  b. More common in males than females.
  c. Always associated with infection.
  d. Inflammation of the renal pelvis.

CHAPTER 14

The Skin

Multiple Choice

1. The surface area of the skin in adults is about:
   a. 0.5–1.0 m².
   b. 1.0–1.5 m².
   c. 1.5–2.0 m².
   d. 2.0–2.5 m².

2. The epidermis:
   a. Is composed of stratified keratinised squamous epithelium.
   b. Lies under the dermis.
   c. Contains nerve endings and blood vessels.
   d. Is replaced every 2 months.

3. The substance mainly responsible for waterproofing the skin is:
   a. Melanin.
   b. Collagen.
   c. Carotene.
   d. Keratin.

4. The dermis:
   a. Contains mast cells.
   b. Consists of areolar tissue and some adipose (fat) tissue.
   c. Contains the openings of sweat glands.
   d. Varies in thickness according to the amount of wear and tear in the area.

5. Pacinian corpuscles are sensory receptors for:
   a. Pain.
   b. Light pressure.
   c. Deep pressure.
   d. Temperature.

6. Sebum is secreted by:
   a. Sweat glands.
   b. Sebaceous glands.
   c. Apocrine glands.
   d. Dermal papillae.

7. Dendritic (Langerhans) cells:
   a. Protect the skin from maceration.
   b. Enable skin hairs to stand erect causing 'goose flesh'.
   c. Assist in regulation of body temperature.
   d. Phagocytose intruding antigens.

8. The substance that affords protection against harmful ultraviolet rays in sunlight is:
  a. Vitamin D.
  b. Interleukin 1.
  c. Sebum.
  d. Melanin.

9. Heat loss:
  a. Occurs by convection when clothes in direct contact with the skin take up heat.
  b. Occurs by evaporation when the body converts sweat to water vapour.
  c. Only occurs though the skin.
  d. Increases when there is vasoconstriction.

10. Heat production is NOT increased when:
  a. Running.
  b. Shivering.
  c. Digesting a meal.
  d. Wearing several layers of clothes.

11. Body temperature:
  a. Is maintained within a fairly constant range to optimise activity of the enzymes needed for metabolism.
  b. Is controlled by the temperature regulating centre in the medulla.
  c. Is under positive feedback control.
  d. Drops in women just after ovulation.

12. In fever:
  a. Vasoconstriction of the arterioles in the skin allows more blood flow there.
  b. The skin is pink in colour and warm to touch.
  c. The temperature regulation centre responds to changes in blood oxygen levels.
  d. Chemicals known as neurotransmitters reset the thermostat in the hypothalamus to a higher level.

13. Hypothermia is defined as core temperature below:
  a. 25°C.
  b. 32°C.
  c. 35°C.
  d. 37°C.

14. In wound healing:
  a. Surgical incisions normally heal by first intention.
  b. Any bacteria present are removed by mast cells.
  c. The first stage is proliferative.
  d. Phagocytes secrete new collagen fibres.

15. An infected open channel that discharges onto the skin is called a:
  a. Fissure.
  b. Fistula.
  c. Scar.
  d. Sinus.

16. Which is not true about older adults?
  a. Reduced vitamin D production predisposes older adults to the effects of demineralisation and reduced bone strength.
  b. As the stratum corneum becomes less active, the epidermis thins.
  c. Fewer elastic and collagen fibres in the dermis leads to wrinkling and sagging.
  d. Temperature regulation becomes less efficient, making older adults more prone to heatstroke and hypothermia.

17. Cold sores are caused by:
  a. Herpes zoster.
  b. Herpes simplex.
  c. *Staphylococcus aureus.*
  d. *Streptococcus pyogenes.*

18. Psoriasis:
  a. Is caused by blockage of sebaceous glands.
  b. Is an infective condition.
  c. Is genetically determined.
  d. Can sometimes be linked to osteoarthritis.

19. Burns:
  a. Are first degree when only the dermis is affected.
  b. Are relatively painless when they are full thickness.
  c. Can heal by first intention when they are full thickness.
  d. May be complicated by hypovolaemic shock when 25% of the body surface is affected.

20. Basal cell carcinoma of the skin:
  a. Is associated with long-term exposure to sunlight.
  b. Is also known as malignant melanoma.
  c. Arises from the walls of lymphatic vessels.
  d. Commonly affects the upper back in males.

CHAPTER 15

Introduction to Immunity

Multiple Choice

1. Specific defence mechanisms, e.g., antibody production, are sometimes called:
a. Innate immunity.
b. Adaptive immunity.
c. Complementary immunity.
d. Immunological surveillance.

2. Which of the following is true of the body's non-specific defences?
a. They include the sweeping clean of epithelial membranes by respiratory cilia and gastrointestinal villi.
b. The skin is an effective barrier and its surface is kept sterile by the secretion of antibacterial sebum.
c. The acidity of urine and vaginal secretions discourages ascending infections of the genitourinary tracts.
d. Lysozyme is an enzyme that keeps the skin supple and waterproof.

3. Complement:
a. Stimulates chemotaxis of phagocytes.
b. Forms part of an immune complex.
c. Is also called immunoglobulin.
d. Is a bacterial protein that stimulates an immune response.

4. What is the acute phase response?
a. The cardinal signs of acute inflammation—pain, swelling, heat and redness.
b. The immune response to infection caused by injury to tissues.
c. Release of systemic inflammatory mediators following tissue damage.
d. Reflex withdrawal of an injured body part from the source of injury.

5. Which of the following inflammatory mediators acts as an endogenous pyrogen, causing fever?
a. Bradykinin.
b. Histamine.
c. Leukotriene.
d. Interleukin.

6. Mycobacteria infections are often resistant to immune defences and produce persistent infections. The best explanation for this is that:
   a. They do not stimulate antibody production.
   b. They tend to cause superficial infections of the skin, relatively inaccessible to defence mechanisms.
   c. They enter host cells and are therefore protected.
   d. They live in the bloodstream, where they can easily evade host defences.

7. Which of the following is NOT associated with adaptive immunity?
   a. Phagocytosis.
   b. Tolerance.
   c. Non-specificity.
   d. Immunological surveillance.

8. Which of the following is true of B-cells but not T-cells?
   a. They are produced in the bone marrow.
   b. They target one specific antigen.
   c. They produce antibodies.
   d. They display tolerance.

9. Antigen presenting cells, such as macrophages:
   a. Are antigen-specific.
   b. Produce antibodies.
   c. Undergo clonal expansion when stimulated by antigen.
   d. Activate T-cells.

10. Regulatory T-cells:
    a. Suppress the immune response.
    b. Are responsible for activating B-cells.
    c. Are the longest-lived subset of T-cells.
    d. Produce antibodies.

11. Exposure to infection stimulates immunity to that infection because, following recovery, the immune individual now has a population of:
    a. Cytotoxic T-cells.
    b. Memory B-cells.
    c. Regulatory T-cells.
    d. Helper T-cells.

12. Antibodies:
    a. Are effective against bacteria, but not bacterial toxins.
    b. Are displayed by B-cells to detect that B-cell's specific antigen.
    c. Are effective in the bloodstream but cannot enter the tissues.
    d. Are albumins.

13. IgA:
    a. Characterises the secondary immune response.
    b. Is often associated with allergy.
    c. Coats membranes and epithelial surfaces.
    d. Is not present in breast milk.

14. The primary immune response is associated with:
   a. Delayed response following antigen exposure.
   b. High levels of IgG.
   c. The presence of memory cells in the circulation.
   d. Viral rather than bacterial infections.

15. Vaccination against a disease gives rise to:
   a. Active natural immunity.
   b. Passive natural immunity.
   c. Passive artificial immunity.
   d. Active artificial immunity.

16. In the immune response, which defence cell increases in numbers in the circulation first?
   a. Macrophage.
   b. Cytotoxic T-cell.
   c. Natural killer cell.
   d. Plasma cell.

17. Reduced numbers of natural killer cells in older age are linked to:
   a. The increased incidence of autoimmune disorders, such as diabetes.
   b. The increased incidence of cancer, as natural killer cells detect and destroy abnormal body cells.
   c. The increased risk of infections, especially respiratory infections.
   d. A reduced number of minor infections, particularly viral infections.

18. Autoimmune disease is an example of:
   a. Type I hypersensitivity.
   b. Type II hypersensitivity.
   c. Type III hypersensitivity.
   d. Type IV hypersensitivity.

19. In HIV infection:
   a. Immune failure and immunodeficiency is a very early feature.
   b. The virus is not detectable in any body fluid except the blood.
   c. The virus produces the enzyme reverse transcriptase to synthesise viral DNA.
   d. The virus has a particular affinity for cells bearing the CD_2 receptor, and establishes itself within these cells, including macrophages and T-helper cells.

20. Which of the following disorders is associated with autoimmunity?
   a. Graves' disease.
   b. Type 2 diabetes.
   c. Osteoarthritis.
   d. Duchenne muscular dystrophy.

CHAPTER 16

The Musculoskeletal System

Multiple Choice

1. Haemopoiesis takes place in the adult skeleton in:
   a. The medullary cavities of limb bones.
   b. Red bone marrow in the epiphyses of long bones.
   c. The diaphyses of long bones.
   d. Spongy bone throughout the skeleton.

2. Which of the following is a sesamoid bone?
   a. The femur.
   b. The first cervical vertebra.
   c. The sternum.
   d. The patella.

3. Which of the following describes the structure of a typical long bone?
   a. The epiphyses are connected by a slender diaphysis.
   b. Yellow bone marrow is found in the spongy bone of the epiphyses.
   c. The marrow cavity is lined with periosteum.
   d. Bone ends that form joints are covered with white fibrocartilage.

4. The major constituent of osteoid is:
   a. Calcium phosphate salts.
   b. Collagen fibres.
   c. Bone cells: osteoblasts and osteoclasts.
   d. Elastic connective tissue.

5. Osteoclasts:
   a. Produce osteoid.
   b. Calcify osteoid.
   c. Demineralise bone.
   d. Ossify cartilage.

6. Which bone cells live in lacunae?
   a. Osteoblasts.
   b. Osteoclasts.
   c. Osteoprogenitor cells.
   d. Osteocytes.

7. Which of the following is found in compact bone tissue but not spongy bone tissue?
   a. A central canal.
   b. Lamellae.
   c. Canaliculi.
   d. Lacunae.

8. Which hormone promotes closure of the epiphyseal growth plate of long bones?
   a. Growth hormone.
   b. Thyroxine.
   c. Testosterone.
   d. Calcitonin.

9. A pathological bone fracture is one that:
   a. Becomes infected.
   b. Is due to existing bone disease.
   c. Fails to heal within an expected timeframe.
   d. Has no clear or understood cause.

10. Osteopenia is caused by:
    a. Excess growth hormone in adults.
    b. Dietary deficiency of calcium in children.
    c. Demineralisation of bone with age.
    d. A genetic tendency for bone fractures.

11. A foramen in a bone is a:
    a. Groove for nerves or blood vessels.
    b. Projection for muscle attachment.
    c. Flat surface for muscle attachment.
    d. A hole through the bone.

12. The adult cranium contains:
    a. Two temporal bones, one frontal bone, two occipital bones and one parietal bone.
    b. One temporal bone, two frontal bones, one occipital bone and two parietal bones.
    c. Two temporal bones, one frontal bone, one occipital bone and two parietal bones.
    d. One temporal bone, one frontal bone, two occipital bones and one parietal bone.

13. Which vitamin is essential for normal mineralisation of bone?
    a. A.
    b. B_1.
    c. C.
    d. D.

14. The appendicular skeleton includes the:
    a. Scapula and clavicle.
    b. Ribs and pelvis.
    c. Clavicle and sternum.
    d. Coccyx and pelvis.

15. The sphenoid bone:
    a. Forms the orbits of the eye.
    b. Is hollowed to accommodate the cerebellum.
    c. Contains the hypophyseal fossa, accommodating the pituitary gland.
    d. Forms the conchae of the nasal cavity.

16. Which of the following is true of the structures called fontanelles?
    a. There are four: the anterior, posterior, mastoid and sphenoidal fontanelles.
    b. They are present at birth, but should have disappeared by the age of 6 weeks.
    c. They are only identifiable by x-ray, and are not detectable in all newborns.
    d. Their function is to prevent any relative movement of the cranial bones during childbirth, to protect the fetal brain.

17. Which of the following is true of the relationship between the atlas and the axis?
   a. The axis sits on top of the atlas, and the bones are held together with a condyloid joint.
   b. The atlas sits on top of the axis, and the transverse ligament holds the dens of the axis in place.
   c. The axis sits on top of the atlas, and the dens of the axis articulates with the occipital bone of the skull.
   d. The atlas sits on top of the axis, and the joint between them permits nodding of the head.

18. How many bones are there in the vertebral column?
   a. 25.
   b. 26.
   c. 27.
   d. 28.

19. The numbers of vertebrae in each section of the vertebral column are:
   a. 8 cervical, 10 thoracic, 5 lumbar, 7 (fused) sacral.
   b. 5 cervical, 12 thoracic, 7 lumbar, 6 (fused) sacral.
   c. 6 cervical, 11 thoracic, 6 lumbar, 5 (fused) sacral.
   d. 7 cervical, 12 thoracic, 5 lumbar, 5 (fused) sacral.

20. Which bone forms joints using its capitulum and trochlea?
   a. Scapula.
   b. Femur.
   c. Humerus.
   d. Tibia.

21. The scaphoid and pisiform bones are found in the:
   a. Wrist.
   b. Cranium.
   c. Vertebral column.
   d. Ankle.

22. Which of the following structures is superior to the others?
   a. Ischial tuberosity.
   b. Symphysis pubis.
   c. Iliac crest.
   d. Acetabulum.

23. How many phalanges are there in the foot?
   a. 12.
   b. 14.
   c. 13.
   d. 15.

24. The pubic symphysis is a:
   a. Synovial joint.
   b. Fibrous joint.
   c. Elastic joint.
   d. Cartilaginous joint.

25. Synovial joints:
   a. Are the only moveable joints of the skeleton.
   b. Include the sutures of the skull.
   c. Are lubricated with a small amount of serous fluid.
   d. Possess a capsule lined with a fibrous ligament.

26. With the arm straight out in front of the body, drawing a circle in the air with the forefinger represents which movement of the arm?
   a. Rotation.
   b. Circumduction.
   c. Extension.
   d. Inversion.

27. Which movement can be made at the interphalangeal joints?
   a. Flexion.
   b. Rotation.
   c. Eversion.
   d. Abduction.

28. The glenoidal labrum stabilises the:
   a. Elbow joint.
   b. Hip joint.
   c. Ankle joint.
   d. Shoulder joint.

29. In rheumatoid arthritis:
   a. There is no genetic component.
   b. 90% of sufferers have rheumatoid factor in the bloodstream.
   c. The first joint to be affected is usually either the knee or hip joint.
   d. Pannus (nodules of connective tissue) may form in the arms.

30. Articular cartilage:
   a. Forms part of the joint sleeve, holding the articulating bones together.
   b. Covers bone surfaces involved in joint formation.
   c. Forms menisci, supporting pads in, e.g. the knee joint.
   d. Encloses the bursae, fluid filled shock absorbers in and around joints.

31. The elbow joint is a:
   a. Condyloid joint.
   b. Saddle joint.
   c. Ball and socket joint.
   d. Hinge joint.

32. How many joints are there between the radius and the ulna?
   a. One.
   b. Two.
   c. Three.
   d. Four.

33. At the wrist, which carpal bones articulate with the radius?
   a. Capitate and scaphoid.
   b. Lunate and hamate.
   c. Triquetrum and hamate.
   d. Scaphoid and lunate.

34. The flexor retinaculum:
   a. Is a large muscle of the forearm, flexing the elbow joint.
   b. Is a tiny muscle of the orbit of the eye.
   c. Is a band of fibrous tissue that forms the carpal tunnel.
   d. Is the most anterior of the vertebral ligaments holding the vertebra together.

35. Within the acetabulum is found the:
   a. Pelvic organs.
   b. Ligamentum teres.
   c. Head of the femur.
   d. Spinal cord.

36. Which bone sits within the quadriceps tendon?
   a. The patella.
   b. The hyoid bone.
   c. The tarsus bone.
   d. The coccyx.

37. The bones contributing to the ankle joint are the:
   a. Talus and tibia.
   b. Calcaneus, tibia and fibula.
   c. Talus, tibia and fibula.
   d. Calcaneus and tibia.

38. Skeletal muscle fibres:
   a. Are branched.
   b. Contract in response to sympathetic stimulation.
   c. Are striated.
   d. Have one, very large, central nucleus.

39. A tendon:
   a. Is formed from the perimysium, epimysium and endomysium of the muscle.
   b. Attaches one bone to another, so is important in stabilising joints.
   c. Is formed of elastic connective tissue.
   d. Is called an aponeurosis when it forms a rope-like band to anchor muscle to bone.

40. Which of the following is stored inside skeletal muscle cells and is essential for cross bridge formation?
   a. Iron.
   b. Sodium.
   c. Oxygen.
   d. Calcium.

41. Within the sarcomere, actin:
   a. Is bound to the Z lines.
   b. Forms the thick filaments.
   c. Crosses the M line.
   d. Is not present in the light bands.

42. The transmitter released at the neuromuscular junction is:
   a. Either noradrenaline or acetylcholine.
   b. Always noradrenaline.
   c. Always acetylcholine.
   d. Usually dopamine.

43. Myasthenia gravis (MG):
   a. Is more common in men than women.
   b. Usually appears between the ages of 20 and 40.
   c. Is caused by a deficiency of acetylcholine.
   d. Causes spasm and rigidity of skeletal muscle.

44. In isometric contraction of skeletal muscle:
   a. The muscle contracts spasmodically and repetitively.
   b. The muscle does not shorten.
   c. Muscle tension does not change.
   d. There is simultaneous contraction of the antagonistic muscle.

45. What is the function of the orbicularis oris muscle?
   a. It raises the eyebrows.
   b. It closes the eyes.
   c. It purses the lips.
   d. It permits smiling.

46. Which large muscle of the back attaches the cervical and thoracic vertebrae to the occipital bone, the scapula and the clavicle, and squares the shoulders?
   a. Trapezius.
   b. Deltoid.
   c. Latissimus dorsi.
   d. Teres major.

47. The linea alba:
   a. Stabilises the vertebral column.
   b. Secures the tarsal bones to the metatarsals.
   c. Gives attachment to the external abdominal obliques.
   d. Is the large, flat tendon of the occipitofrontalis.

48. The main flexor of the elbow joint is the:
   a. Biceps brachii.
   b. Flexor carpi radialis.
   c. Triceps brachii.
   d. Brachialis.

49. Which of the following is NOT a member of the quadriceps femoris group of muscles?
   a. Vastus lateralis.
   b. Vastus medialis.
   c. Vastus intermedius.
   d. Vastus superioris.

50. The gastrocnemius:
   a. Lies deep to the soleus.
   b. Is one of the hamstring muscles.
   c. Has two heads, originating on the femur.
   d. Is the longest muscle in the body.

CHAPTER 17

Genetics

Multiple Choice

1. The functional units of DNA are called:
a. Chromosomes.
b. Alleles.
c. Genomes.
d. Genes.

2. Chromosomes:
a. Come in pairs, numbered from 1–46.
b. Possess end regions called telomeres, which accumulate additional DNA with age.
c. Are different sizes: chromosome pair 1 is bigger than chromosome pair 10.
d. Are only seen in resting cells that are neither preparing to divide nor actively dividing.

3. Which of the following could be a nucleotide of DNA?
a. Deoxyribose sugar, adenine base, phosphate group.
b. Either deoxyribose or ribose sugar, cytosine base, phosphate group.
c. Deoxyribose sugar, thiamine base, phosphate group.
d. Deoxyribose sugar, uracil base, phosphate group.

4. What distinguishes the male sex chromosomes from the female?
a. They comprise two short Y chromosomes.
b. There is one X chromosome and one Y chromosome, and the X is larger than the Y.
c. They comprise two X chromosomes, but one is much shorter than the other.
d. They comprise two Y chromosomes, which are larger than the X chromosome.

5. Which of the following heritable disorders is due to possession of an extra chromosome?
a. Cri-du-chat syndrome.
b. Phenylketonuria.
c. Down's syndrome.
d. Cystic fibrosis.

6. In complementary base pairing:
a. Uracil always pairs with thymine.
b. Cytosine always pairs with adenine.
c. Guanine always pairs with uracil.
d. Thymine always pairs with adenine.

7. In addition to the nucleus, which organelle contains DNA?
a. the mitochondrion.
b. The endoplasmic reticulum.
c. The Golgi apparatus.
d. The centrosome.

8. Messenger RNA:
   a. Is produced by ribosomes in the cytoplasm.
   b. Is synthesised during the process of translation.
   c. Is built of base triplets, which code for individual amino acids.
   d. Binds directly to a gene to activate or deactivate it.

9. On average, how many amino acids are used to produce proteins in humans?
   a. 15.
   b. 20.
   c. 25.
   d. 30.

10. Which of the following cells is haploid?
   a. Erythrocyte.
   b. Zygote.
   c. Neurone.
   d. Ovum.

11. Meiosis:
   a. Involves three distinct cell divisions to produce gametes.
   b. Ensures the daughter cells have exact copies of the parent cell's DNA.
   c. Produces four haploid daughter cells, all genetically different to each other.
   d. Involves the process of crossing over, which takes place at the second meiotic division.

12. The tongue rolling gene has two forms, T and t. Which of the following is true?
   a. If both forms are present in an individual, he or she is said to be homozygous.
   b. The genotype tt is said to be heterozygous recessive.
   c. Individuals with genotype TT have a non-tongue rolling phenotype.
   d. Both homozygous dominant and heterozygous individuals are tongue rollers.

13. Homozygous alleles are:
   a. Two identical copies of the same gene on matching chromosomal loci.
   b. Two identical copies of the same chromosome, following mitosis.
   c. Two identical chromatids belonging to the same chromosome.
   d. Either of the chromosomes belonging to a chromosome pair.

14. If both parents are heterozygous for a particular gene, which of the following is true of their potential children?
   a. They would all be heterozygous for the gene.
   b. They would all be homozygous for the gene.
   c. Statistically, 25% of their children would be heterozygous for the gene.
   d. Statistically, 50% of their children would be homozygous for the gene.

15. For the same gene as in question 14, the father is heterozygous and the mother is homozygous recessive. If they have four children, which of the following represents the statistical likelihood of their genetic makeup?
   a. One homozygous recessive child, one homozygous dominant child and two heterozygous children.
   b. Two homozygous recessive children and two heterozygous children.
   c. Two homozygous dominant children and two heterozygous children.
   d. One homozygous dominant child and three heterozygous children.

16. Which of the following couples could NOT produce a child with blood group O?
a. Mother blood group AB, father blood group O.
b. Mother blood group B, father blood group B.
c. Mother blood group A, father blood group B.
d. Mother blood group O, father blood group A.

17. Which of the following is true of sex-linked inheritance?
a. Daughters cannot inherit a sex-linked gene.
b. A sex-linked gene is carried on the Y chromosome.
c. Males have only one copy of a sex-linked gene.
d. Sex-linked genes are transmitted by the father, not the mother.

18. If a father is colour blind, and the mother has two normal copies of the colour vision gene, which of the following children could be born?
a. A carrier daughter.
b. A colour blind son.
c. A carrier son.
d. A homozygous daughter with normal colour vision.

19. A mutation in DNA:
a. Invariably leads to the development of cancer.
b. Is an irreversible change to DNA structure.
c. Is not hereditable, i.e. is not passed from parent to child.
d. Can trigger destruction of the affected cell by the immune system.

20. In Klinefelter syndrome:
a. Both sexes are equally affected.
b. The gene responsible is carried on the X chromosome.
c. Intelligence is usually impaired.
d. Fertility is normal.

CHAPTER 18

The Reproductive System

Multiple Choice

1. Which of the following is part of the female external genitalia?
a. Vestibular glands.
b. Cervix.
c. Perineum.
d. Mons pubis.

2. The space between the labia minora is the:
a. Hymen.
b. Perineum.
c. Vestibule.
d. Symphysis pubis.

3. The normal uterus:
a. Is anteverted.
b. Is inferior to the urinary bladder.
c. Lies posteriorly to the vesicouterine pouch.
d. Is lateral to the rectum.

4. Which of the following is true of the vagina?
a. The anterior wall is longer than the posterior wall.
b. The uterine cervix projects into its distal end.
c. It possesses no secretory glands in its epithelium
d. The rugae formed in its walls aid sperm movement.

5. Which surface of the uterus is NOT covered with peritoneum?
a. The superior fundus.
b. The posterior body.
c. The anterior fundus.
d. The lateral body.

6. The basal layer of the uterine wall lies between:
a. The functional layer and the perimetrium.
b. The myometrium and the functional layer.
c. The endometrium and the perimetrium.
d. The perimetrium and the myometrium.

7. The thickest layer of the uterine wall is the:
a. Perimetrium.
b. Myometrium.
c. Endometrium.
d. Mesometrium.

8. What is the function of the round ligament?
a. It attaches the uterus to the labia majora.
b. It is a flat sheet folded over the upper uterus and uterine tubes.
c. It secures the posterior cervix and vagina to the sacrum.
d. It secures the cervix and vagina to the pelvic walls.

9. The organism responsible for which of the following sexually transmitted infections also causes trachoma, a serious eye infection?
a. Syphilis.
b. HIV/AIDS.
c. Chlamydia.
d. Gonorrhoea.

10. What is the definition of an embryo?
a. The fertilised egg before it implants in the uterine wall.
b. The developmental stage of the 4 weeks after implantation.
c. The developmental stage until the placenta has fully formed.
d. The first 8 weeks of development after fertilisation.

11. The fimbriae of the uterine tubes:
a. Line the tubes to propel the ovum towards the uterus.
b. Are not enclosed in the broad ligament, but open into the peritoneal cavity.
c. Form a trumpet-like structure at the proximal end of each uterine tube.
d. Are the usual site of fertilisation.

12. Which of the following is true of the ovary?
a. Its outer layer, the cortex, contains the primordial follicles.
b. It is attached to the uterus by the mesovarium.
c. The inner medullary tissue is responsible for secretion of oestrogens.
d. It has no lymphatic drainage.

13. The female gonadotrophins:
a. Are secreted by the ovary.
b. Are released from the hypothalamus.
c. Include luteinising hormone (LH).
d. Include oestrogen.

14. During the first half of the female reproductive cycle, a surge in which hormone(s) trigger(s) ovulation?
a. Progesterone.
b. Follicle stimulating hormone (FSH).
c. Oestrogen and progesterone.
d. LH.

15. The secretory phase of the female reproductive cycle is associated with:
a. Menstruation.
b. Peaks of oestrogen and progesterone secretion.
c. Rising levels of FSH.
d. The development of one or more ovarian follicles.

16. After ovulation, high blood levels of oestrogen and progesterone:
a. Suppress the anterior pituitary and keep FSH levels low.
b. Trigger follicular development in the ovarian cortex.
c. Inhibit development of the uterine lining.
d. Stimulate the production of LH to support the corpus luteum.

17. Which of the following is characteristic of the female menopause?
a. Thinning and coarsening of the skin.
b. Enlargement of the breasts.
c. Rising blood cholesterol levels.
d. Falling levels of LH and FSH.

18. Which hormone promotes milk release in the lactating breast?
a. Oestrogen.
b. Prolactin.
c. Progesterone.
d. Oxytocin.

19. Which of the following is a protective factor in breast cancer?
a. Multiple pregnancies.
b. Late menopause.
c. Increasing age.
d. Early onset of puberty.

20. What is the male equivalent of the female ovary?
a. Scrotum.
b. Penis.
c. Testis.
d. Epididymis.

21. Which structures are linked by the deferent duct?
a. The seminal duct and the urethra.
b. The epididymis and the ejaculatory duct.
c. The prostatic duct and the seminal duct.
d. The urethra and the ejaculatory duct.

22. The optimal temperature for spermatogenesis is:
a. 38°C.
b. 37°C.
c. 36°C.
d. 34°C.

23. Which of the following represents the path of sperm from the testis to the exterior?
a. Deferent duct, epididymis, urethra, ejaculatory duct.
b. Ejaculatory duct, deferent duct, epididymis, urethra.
c. Epididymis, deferent duct, ejaculatory duct, urethra.
d. Deferent duct, epididymis, ejaculatory duct, urethra.

24. Seminal fluid:
a. Comprises 60% of sperm volume.
b. Is produced by the prostate gland.
c. Is a thin, watery fluid.
d. Is slightly acidic to neutralise the alkalinity of the vagina.

25. Which of the following is true of the corpora cavernosa of the penis?
    a. They form the bulb of the penis.
    b. They are the lateral columns of erectile tissue.
    c. They enclose the urethra.
    d. They form the prepuce of the penis.

26. When ejaculated at orgasm, sperm pass through the male reproductive passageways due to:
    a. Ciliary action.
    b. Gravity.
    c. Peristalsis.
    d. Propulsion by the spermatozoal tail.

27. A blastocyst:
    a. Is a non-malignant tumour of the ovary.
    b. Is the structure that nourishes the developing fetus prior to placental maturity.
    c. Is the functional unit in the testis in which spermatozoa are produced.
    d. Is an early embryo of between 70 and 100 cells implanted in the uterine wall.

28. The commonest cause of scrotal swelling is:
    a. A testicular tumour.
    b. Hydrocele.
    c. Cryptorchidism.
    d. Epididymitis.

29. Which of the following is seen in the developing embryo at about 3 months of gestation?
    a. Blood cell formation starts.
    b. Presence of a clearly defined respiratory tree.
    c. A beating heart.
    d. The appearance of limb buds.

30. In fetal development, ossification of the skeleton begins at:
    a. 1 month.
    b. 2 months.
    c. 3 months.
    d. 4 months.

CHAPTER 1

Anatomy and Organisation of the Body

Feedback

1.
  a. False. Physiology is the study of how the body systems work and the ways in which their integrated activities maintain the life and health of the individual.
  b. False. Pathology is the study of abnormalities.
  c. **Correct.** Anatomy is the study of the structure of the body and the physical relationships between its constituent parts.
  d. False. Pathophysiology considers how the abnormalities affect body functions, often causing illness.
  REF: Page 1

2.
  a. False. Cells with similar structure and functions are found together in complex organisms, forming tissues.
  b. **Correct.** Cells are the smallest independent units of living matter and there are trillions of them within the body.
  c. False. Organs are made from a number of different types of tissues.
  d. False. Systems consist of a number of organs and tissues that together contribute to one or more survival needs of the body.
  REF: Page 2

3.
  a. False. The special senses provide information about the external environment.
  b. False. The respiratory system is involved in intake of raw materials and elimination of waste.
  c. False. The reproductive system enables survival of the human species.
  d. **Correct.** The endocrine system responds to changes in the internal environment to maintain homeostasis.
  REF: Pages 3 and 34

4.
  a. True. The blood transports substances around the body.
  b. True. The lymphatic system carries lymph through a network of lymph vessels.
  c. **Correct.** The nervous system is a rapid communication system.
  d. True. The cardiovascular system consists of a network of blood vessels and the heart.
  REF: Page 3

5.
   a. False.
   b. False.
   c. **Correct.** In adults, the body contains about 5–6 L of blood.
   d. False.
   REF: Page 4

6.
   a. True. Plasma is mainly water with a wide range of substances dissolved or suspended in it.
   b. **Correct.** Chromosomes are found in the nuclei of cells, not in the blood.
   c. True. Platelets are the tiny cell fragments essential for blood clotting.
   d. True. Erythrocytes (red blood cells) carry oxygen and some carbon dioxide between body cells and the lungs.
   REF: Page 4

7.
   a. True. Erythrocytes are the red blood cells.
   b. True. Leukocytes are the white blood cells.
   c. True. Platelets, or thrombocytes, are tiny cell fragments present in blood.
   d. **Correct.** Adipocytes (fat cells) are not present in blood.
   REF: Pages 4 and 51

8.
   a. **Correct.** Red blood cells transport oxygen and, to a lesser extent, carbon dioxide between the lungs and all body cells.
   b. False. White blood cells are mainly concerned with protecting the body against infection.
   c. False. Platelets play an essential part in blood clotting.
   d. False. Red blood cells are smaller than white blood cells.
   REF: Page 4

9.
   a. **Correct.** Lymphatics, or lymph vessels, are part of the lymphatic system that transports lymph.
   b. Arteries carry blood away from the heart.
   c. Veins return blood to the heart.
   d. Capillaries link the arteries and veins.
   REF: Page 4

10.
   a. False. Capillary walls are only one cell thick.
   b. **Correct.** They enable exchange of substances, e.g., nutrients, oxygen and cellular waste products, between blood and body tissues.
   c. False. The smallest vessels of the lymphatic system are known as lymphatic capillaries.
   d. False. Capillaries transport blood between the arteries and veins.
   REF: Page 4

11.
   a. **Correct.** The pulmonary circulation transports blood to and from the lungs.
   b. False. The systemic circulation transports blood to and from cells in all other parts of the body except the lungs.
   c. False. Lymph does travel towards the point where it joins the bloodstream near the heart, but this is not the pulmonary circulation.
   d. False. Lymph is not transported to or from the lungs.
   REF: Page 5

12.
    a. **Correct.** The heart is a muscular sac with four chambers.
    b. False. The heart receives blood returning from the body through veins.
    c. False. The heart beats between 65 and 75 times per minute at rest.
    d. False. The heart muscle is not under conscious (voluntary) control.
    REF: Page 5

13.
    a. False. Transport in the lymphatic system starts in tiny blind-ended lymphatic capillaries which become larger and transport lymph through a series of lymph nodes, eventually draining the lymph through large lymphatics into the bloodstream.
    b. False. The pores in the walls of lymph capillaries are larger than those of the blood capillaries.
    c. **Correct.**
    d. False. There are sites for formation and maturation of lymphocytes (not erythrocytes).
    REF: Page 5

14.
    a. False.
    b. **Correct.** Reflex actions are fast, involuntary and usually protective motor responses to specific stimuli.
    c. False.
    d. False.
    REF: Page 6

15.
    a. False.
    b. False.
    c. **Correct.** Pain is not one of the special senses.
    d. False. Smell, sight and balance are all special senses.
    REF: Figure 1.8, page 7

16.
    a. False. Endocrine glands are discrete and situated in different parts of the body, but they have no connections.
    b. False. Changes in blood hormone levels are generally controlled by negative feedback mechanisms.
    c. **Correct.** Endocrine glands synthesise and secrete hormones.
    d. False. The responses that control body functions are slower but more precise than those of the nervous system.
    REF: Page 6

17.
    a. **Correct.** The liver is an accessory organ of the digestive system.
    b. False.
    c. False.
    d. False. The rectum, pharynx and stomach are parts of the digestive tract and are therefore accessory organs.
    REF: Page 8

18.
  a. False. Gas exchange does not take place in the trachea.
  b. False. Gas exchange does not take place in the bronchi (although it does take place in the smallest bronchioles).
  c. False. Gas exchange does not take place in the bronchi.
  d. **Correct.** The alveoli are surrounded by a network of tiny capillaries and are the sites where vital gas exchange between the lungs and the blood takes place.
  REF: Page 7

19.
  a. False. Anabolism is building or synthesising large and complex substances.
  b. False. Catabolism is breaking down substances.
  c. **Correct.** Metabolism is the sum total of the chemical activity in the body. It consists of anabolism and catabolism.
  d. False. Homeostasis is the maintenance of a stable internal environment.
  REF: Pages 8 and 34

20.
  a. **Correct.** A fertilised egg.
  b. False. A female gamete is known as an ovum.
  c. False. A male gamete is known as a spermatozoon.
  d. False. A fertilised egg must undergo considerable development before it becomes a fetus in the 11th week of pregnancy.
  REF: Page 10

21.
  a. False. Anterior describes a structure being nearer to the front of the body.
  b. **Correct.** Medial describes a structure being nearer to the midline.
  c. False. Lateral describes a structure being further from the midline or at the side of the body.
  d. False. Superior describes a structure being nearer to the head.
  REF: Page 11, Table 1.2

22.
  a. False. The head is referred to as cephalic.
  b. False. The navel is referred to as umbilical.
  c. **Correct.** The arm is referred to as brachial.
  d. False. The leg is referred to as crural.
  REF: Page 12, Figure 1.16

23.
  a. False.
  b. False.
  c. False. The skull, vertebral column and ribs are part of the axial skeleton.
  d. **Correct.** The shoulder girdle is part of the appendicular skeleton, not the axial skeleton.
  REF: Page 13

24.
  a. False.
  b. False.
  c. **Correct.** The mandible or lower jaw is the only movable bone of the skull.
  d. False. The frontal bone, maxilla and temporal bones are not movable.
  REF: Page 13

25.
   a. False.
   b. False.
   c. **Correct.** The thoracic cage gives attachment to intercostal muscles, which move the ribs during respiration.
   d. False.
   REF: Page 14

26.
   a. False. The peritoneum is the epithelial lining of abdominal cavity that also covers many abdominal organs.
   b. **Correct.** The mediastinum is the space between the lungs, including the structures found there, such as the heart, oesophagus and blood vessels.
   c. False. The pericardium is the epithelial lining of the pericardial cavity that also surrounds the heart.
   d. False. The thoracic cavity is a cavity whose boundaries are formed by the thoracic cage and associated muscles.
   REF: Pages 17 and 271, Figure 10.13C

27.
   a. False. The hypogastric region is one of the nine regions of abdominal cavity.
   b. False. The left iliac fossa is one of the nine regions of abdominal cavity.
   c. False. The hypochondriac region is one of the nine regions of abdominal cavity.
   d. **Correct.** The diaphragm is not a region of abdominal cavity. It forms the superior boundary of abdominal cavity, separating it from thoracic cavity.
   REF: Page 18, Figure 1.26

28.
   a. False. Aetiology is the cause of a disease.
   b. **Correct.** Pathogenesis is the nature of the disease process and its effect on normal body functioning.
   c. False. Complications are other consequences that might arise if the disease progresses.
   d. False. Prognosis is the likely outcome.
   REF: Page 23, Box 1.1

29.
   a. **Correct.** Inflammation is a tissue response to any kind of tissue damage, such as trauma or infection.
   b. False. Abnormal immune responses arise when the normally protective immune system causes undesirable effects.
   c. False. Thrombosis is the effect and consequence of abnormal changes in the blood and/or blood vessel walls.
   d. False. Degeneration is structural deterioration of tissue, causing impaired function.
   REF: Page 23

30.
   a. False. An acquired disorder develops any time after birth.
   b. False. A communicable disease can be transmitted (spread) from one individual to another.
   c. **Correct.** An iatrogenic condition results from a healthcare intervention.
   d. False. A syndrome is a collection of signs and symptoms that tend to occur together.
   REF: Page 23, Box 1.2

CHAPTER 2

Physiological Chemistry and Processes

Feedback

1.
a. False. The definition of an element is a substance containing only ONE type of atom.
b. False. The definition of a compound is a substance containing more than one type of element.
c. **Correct.** Water is a compound containing hydrogen and oxygen.
d. False. The body is composed almost entirely of only four types of atom: carbon, hydrogen, oxygen and nitrogen.
REF: Page 29

2.
a. False. Electrons are negatively charged but have nearly no mass and orbit the nucleus.
b. **Correct.**
c. False. Only protons and neutrons are found in the atomic nucleus.
d. False. The sum of protons and neutrons is called the atomic weight.
REF: Page 28

3.
a. **Correct.**
b. False. Sodium has eleven protons, twelve neutrons and eleven electrons.
c. False. Potassium has nineteen protons, twenty neutrons and nineteen electrons.
d. False. Carbon has six protons, six neutrons and six electrons.
REF: Page 28

4.
a. False.
b. False.
c. False.
d. **Correct.** The two isotopes of chlorine have atomic weights of 35 and 37. Most chlorine atoms have an atomic weight of 35, so the average atomic weight is only 35.5.
REF: Page 28

5.
a. **Correct.** The ideal electron numbers for the first three electron shells, from the nucleus out, are two, eight and eighteen. When the shells are full, the atom is stable.
b. False.
c. False.
d. False.
REF: Page 28

6.
   a. False. The bond is ionic.
   b. False. There is one sodium atom and one chloride atom.
   c. **Correct.**
   d. False. Ionic bonds are fairly weak and easily disrupted.
   REF: Page 29

7.
   a. False.
   b. **Correct.**
   c. False.
   d. False.
   REF: Page 30, Table 2.2

8.
   a. False. Breast milk usually has a pH of about 6.
   b. False. Gastric fluids are usually between pH 1 and 2.
   c. False. Saliva is usually acid, as low as pH 5.4, to activate salivary amylase.
   d. **Correct.** Blood pH is between 7.35 and 7.45.
   REF: Page 30, Figure 2.6

9.
   a. **Correct.**
   b. False. Proteins contain oxygen, carbon, hydrogen and nitrogen, as well as other elements such as sulphur, magnesium and zinc.
   c. False. Lipids contain carbon, hydrogen and oxygen, but less oxygen than in carbohydrates.
   d. False. Nucleotides contain phosphate and nitrogen as well as oxygen, carbon and hydrogen.
   REF: Page 32

10.
   a. False.
   b. **Correct.**
   c. False.
   d. False.
   REF: Page 33, Figure 2.10

11.
   a. False.
   b. False.
   c. **Correct.**
   d. False.
   REF: Page 33

12.
   a. False. ATP releases energy when it is broken down, but oxygen is not required for this.
   b. False. ATP is synthesised from ADP in the mitochondria by adding a phosphate group to ADP.
   c. False. Oxygen is (usually) used to produce ATP, but ATP releases water, energy and a phosphate group when it is broken down.
   d. **Correct.**
   REF: Page 34

13.
  a. False. This describes a catabolic (breaking down) reaction.
  b. **Correct.**
  c. False. Enzymes greatly increase the rate of biochemical reactions.
  d. False. One or more substrates enter the reaction and bind to the active site on the enzyme, and products, not substrates, are released.
  REF: Page 34
14.
  a. **Correct.**
  b. False.
  c. False.
  d. False.
  REF: Page 34
15.
  a. False.
  b. False.
  c. **Correct.**
  d. False.
  REF: Page 36
16.
  a. False.
  b. False.
  c. **Correct.**
  d. False.
  REF: Page 38, Figure 2.13
17.
  a. False. Osmosis is passive (requires no energy).
  b. False. Osmosis is specifically the movement of water molecules.
  c. **Correct.** The cell membrane is freely permeable to water.
  d. False. During osmosis, water molecules move down their concentration gradient.
  REF: Page 37
18.
  a. **Correct.** Diffusion is passive (requires no energy).
  b. False. Diffusion can occur across a semipermeable membrane, but also refers to distribution of molecules evenly throughout a solution.
  c. False. Many biological molecules are too big or too heavily charged to diffuse across the cell membrane.
  d. False. Without energy, molecules can only diffuse down their concentration gradient.
  REF: Page 38
19.
  a. False.
  b. False.
  c. False.
  d. **Correct.**
  REF: Page 38
20.
  a. False.
  b. **Correct.**
  c. False.
  d. False.
  REF: Page 38

CHAPTER 3

Cells and Tissues

Feedback

1.
   a. False.
   b. False.
   c. **Correct.** The plasma membrane consists of a bilayer of phospholipids with the hydrophilic heads facing outwards.
   d. False.
   REF: Page 42

2.
   a. False. Receptors for hormones and other chemical messengers are associated with membrane proteins, not carbohydrates.
   b. **Correct.** Branched carbohydrate molecules attached to some cell membrane surface proteins give the cell its immunological identity.
   c. False. Transmembrane proteins form the water-filled channels that allow very small, water-soluble ions to cross the membrane.
   d. False. Enzymes are made from protein.
   REF: Page 42

3.
   a. False.
   b. **Correct.** The plasma membrane is selectively permeable.
   c. False.
   d. False.
   REF: Page 43

4.
   a. **Correct.** The sodium-potassium pump is a form of active transport and therefore requires energy.
   b. False.
   c. False.
   d. False. Osmosis, facilitated diffusion and diffusion are all forms of passive transport and, as such, do not require energy.
   REF: Pages 43 and 44

5.
   a. False. Facilitated diffusion enables small molecules to cross plasma membranes.
   b. False. Diffusion enables small molecules to cross plasma membranes.
   c. False. In osmosis, only water molecules cross plasma membranes.
   d. **Correct.** Pinocytosis and phagocytosis are bulk transport mechanisms that transport particulate materials across plasma membranes into cells.
   REF: Pages 43 and 44, Figure 3.5

6.
  a. False. Skeletal muscle fibres contain several nuclei.
  b. **Correct.** All body cells have nuclei, with the exception of mature erythrocytes (red blood cells).
  c. False. White blood cells contain single nuclei.
  d. False. Columnar epithelial cells contain single nuclei.
  REF: Page 44

7.
  a. and b. False. When a cell prepares to divide, the DNA forms distinct structures in the nucleus called chromatids.
  c. **Correct.** In the non-dividing cell, DNA is present as a fine network of threads called chromatin.
  d. False. The nucleolus is a spherical structure within the nucleus.
  REF: Page 44

8.
  a. False. Mitochondria are small, membranous, sausage-shaped structures described as the power house of the cell.
  b. **Correct.** The nucleus is the largest organelle.
  c. False. Ribosomes are tiny granules composed of RNA and protein.
  d. False. Lysosomes are small, membranous vesicles.
  REF: Page 44

9.
  a. **Correct.** Synthesis of lipids and steroid hormones is a function of smooth endoplasmic reticulum.
  b. False.
  c. False.
  d. False.
  REF: Page 45

10.
  a. False.
  b. False.
  c. False. Smooth endoplasmic reticulum, the Golgi apparatus and lysosomes are all membranous organelles.
  d. **Correct.** The centrosome is made from a pair of microtubules (protein fibres) and plays an important role in cell division.
  REF: Page 46

11.
  a. False. The cytoskeleton is an extensive network of protein fibres.
  b. **Correct.** Flagella are the single, long, whip-like projections containing microtubules that form the tails of spermatozoa.
  c. False. Microvilli are tiny projections that cover the exposed surface of certain types of cells.
  d. False. Cilia are microscopic hair-like projections along the free borders of some cells.
  REF: Page 46

12.
a. **False.** Mitosis is the phase of the cell cycle resulting in two new, genetically identical daughter cells.
b. **False.** Meiosis is the process that leads to the formation of gametes, i.e., ova and spermatozoa.
c. **False.** The cell cycle includes mitosis and interphase.
d. **Correct.** Interphase consists of three stages and is the period between cell divisions.
REF: Page 46

13.
a. **False.** G_1 phase is the first gap phase of interphase where the cell grows in size and volume.
b. **Correct.** G_0 phase is not part of interphase, as some cells do not continue to another round of the cell cycle, but instead enter a resting phase (G_0).
c. **False.** Synthesis of DNA (during the S phase) is part of interphase.
d. **False.** G_2 phase is the second gap phase where the cell grows further and prepares for division.
REF: Page 46, Figure 3.10

14.
a. **Correct.** The mitotic apparatus appears in prophase and consists of two centrioles separated by the mitotic spindle.
b. **False.** The chromatids align on the centre of the spindle in metaphase.
c. **False.** The chromosomes migrate to each end of spindle in anaphase.
d. **False.** The mitotic spindle disappears in telophase.
REF: Figure 3.11

15.
a. **False.** The trachea is lined with ciliated columnar epithelium.
b. **False.** The stomach is lined with columnar epithelium containing glands.
c. **False.** The bladder is lined with transitional epithelium.
d. **Correct.** The heart is lined with squamous epithelium, known as the endocardium.
REF: Page 48

16.
a. **False.** Columnar epithelium lines many internal organs and is often adapted to suit its function, e.g., in the stomach, small intestine and trachea.
b. **Correct.** Keratinised stratified squamous epithelium is found on dry surfaces subjected to wear and tear, e.g., the skin, hair and nails.
c. **False.** Nonkeratinised stratified squamous epithelium protects moist surfaces subjected to wear and tear, e.g., the conjunctiva of eyes, the lining of the mouth, the pharynx, the oesophagus and the vagina.
d. **False.** Transitional epithelium lines several parts of the urinary tract, including the bladder.
REF: Page 49

17.
a. False.
b. False.
c. **Correct.** Transitional epithelium lines the bladder, and its arrangement allows it to stretch as it fills with urine.
d. False.
REF: Page 49

18.

    a. False. Fibroblasts are found in connective tissue, where they manufacture collagen and elastic fibres.

    b. False. Fat cells or adipocytes occur in many types of connective tissue and are especially abundant in adipose tissue.

    c. False. Leukocytes or white blood cells are normally found in small numbers in healthy connective tissue, but they migrate in significant numbers during infection.

    d. **Correct.** Erythrocytes are not present in connective tissue.

    REF: Page 50

19.

    a. **Correct.** Reticular tissue contains reticular cells and white blood cells and is found in lymph nodes and lymph glands.

    b. False. Fibrous tissue is found in, e.g., ligaments and muscle fasciae.

    c. False. Elastic tissue in found in, e.g., the walls of large blood vessels and the trachea and bronchi, where it enables stretching when required.

    d. False. Elastic fibrocartilage provides structures with shape and support. It is found in, e.g., the ear and epiglottis.

    REF: Page 51

20.

    a. True. Kupffer cells in the liver sinusoids are part of the monocyte-macrophage (mononuclear phagocyte) defence system.

    b. True. Sinus-lining cells in the lymph nodes and spleen are part of the monocyte-macrophage (mononuclear phagocyte) defence system.

    c. True. Microglial cells in the brain are part of the monocyte-macrophage (mononuclear phagocyte) defence system.

    d. **Correct.** All of the above are parts of the monocyte-macrophage (mononuclear phagocyte) defence system.

    REF: Page 50

21.

    a. False. Hyaline cartilage is found covering the ends of long bones and in the trachea and bronchi.

    b. False. Elastic fibrocartilage is found in the pinna of ear and in the epiglottis.

    c. **Correct.** Fibrocartilage is found in intervertebral discs and in the semilunar cartilage of knee joint.

    d. False. Fibrous tissue is not found in the intervertebral discs.

    REF: Page 53

22.

    a. **Correct.** Some smooth muscle has the intrinsic ability to initiate its own contractions (has automaticity), e.g., peristalsis.

    b. False.

    c. False.

    d. False. Automaticity is not a property of skeletal muscles, neurones or glial cells.

    REF: Pages 53 and 54

23.

    a. False. Neurones cannot regenerate, as they are unable to divide.

    b. **Correct.** Cuboidal epithelium cells can regenerate.

    c. False. Skeletal muscle cells cannot regenerate, as they are unable to divide.

    d. False.

    REF: Page 55

24.
  a. False. Synovial membrane lines synovial joints but is an epithelial membrane.
  b. False. The peritoneum is the epithelial membrane that lines the abdominal cavity and surrounds many abdominal organs.
  c. False. The pleura is the epithelial membrane that lines the thoracic cavity and surrounds the lungs.
  d. **Correct.** The pericardium is the epithelial membrane that lines the pericardial cavity and surrounds the heart.
  REF: Page 55

25.
  a. False. Glands are made from epithelial tissue.
  b. False. Endocrine glands release their secretions (hormones) into the bloodstream.
  c. **Correct.** Exocrine glands are classified as simple or compound, depending on their complexity.
  d. False. Exocrine glands do not secrete hormones. Their secretions include, e.g., mucus, saliva and earwax.
  REF: Page 55, Figure 3.27

26.
  a. False. Hyperplasia occurs when cells divide more quickly than normal, increasing in number and increasing the size of the tissue, e.g., the glandular milk-producing tissue of the breasts during lactation.
  b. False. Hypertrophy occurs when cells within a tissue enlarge in response to additional demands, e.g., skeletal muscle in response to fitness training.
  c. False. Necrosis is cell death resulting from lack of oxygen.
  d. **Correct.** Apoptosis is normal genetically programmed death of cells at the end of their natural lifespan.
  REF: Page 56

27.
  a. False. A sarcoma arises from connective tissue.
  b. **Correct.** An adenoma arises from glandular tissue.
  c. False. A myoma arises from muscle tissue.
  d. False. An osteoma arises from bone tissue.
  REF: Page 57

28.
  a. True.
  b. True.
  c. True.
  d. **Correct.** The statements above are all true.
  REF: Page 57

29.
  a. False. Malignant tumours typically have poorly differentiated cells.
  b. False. Malignant tumours may spread locally.
  c. **Correct.** Benign tumours are usually encapsulated.
  d. False. Malignant tumours are associated with metastases.
  REF: Page 57, Table 3.1

30.
   a. False. Bronchial tumours commonly spread to the adrenal glands and brain.
   b. False. Tumours of the digestive system commonly spread to the liver though the hepatic portal circulation.
   c. False. Prostate and thyroid tumours commonly spread to the pelvic bones.
   d. **Correct.** Breast tumours commonly spread to the vertebrae, bone and brain.
   REF: Page 58, Table 3.2

CHAPTER 4

The Blood

Feedback

1.
  a. False.
  b. False.
  c. **Correct.**
  d. False
  REF: Figure 4.1

2.
  a. False.
  b. **Correct.**
  c. False.
  d. False.
  REF: Page 62

3.
  a. **Correct.** Transferrin is an albumin that transports iron in the blood.
  b. and d. False. Thyroglobulin and immunoglobulin are globulins.
  c. False. Fibrinogen is the most abundant clotting protein in plasma, and represents the third most abundant plasma protein after the albumins and the globulins.
  REF: Page 62

4.
  a. **Correct.** Anaemia is a general term, and can be caused by various factors, including b, c and d.
  b. False.
  c. False.
  d. False.
  REF: Page 73

5.
  a. False. Erythropoiesis is specifically the production of red blood cells.
  b. False. Haemosynthesis is not a term used in biology.
  c. False. Leukocytosis means an increased white blood cell count.
  d. **Correct.** Haemopoiesis is the general term for the production of blood cells and platelets.
  REF: Figure 4.3

6.
   a. False. They are biconcave discs, meaning the central portion is thinner than the outer portion.
   b. False. They contain very few organelles (a few mitochondria for energy) and no nucleus.
   c. **Correct.**
   d. False. Their membranes are flexible, so that they can deform to squeeze through narrow capillaries: red blood cells do not leave the bloodstream unless blood vessel walls are damaged.
   REF: Page 63

7.
   a. **Correct.**
   b. False.
   c. False.
   d. False.
   REF: Page 65

8.
   a. False. Metabolically active tissues tend to have lower pH values due to increased waste production, and therefore need more oxygen.
   b. False. Metabolically active tissues consume more oxygen than normal, and therefore need more oxygen.
   c. **Correct.** Cooler temperatures, such as those found in the lungs, tend to promote oxygen and haemoglobin binding rather than release.
   d. False. Metabolically active tissues produce more carbon dioxide than normal, and therefore need more oxygen.
   REF: Page 66

9.
   a. False. Erythropoiesis takes about 7 days.
   b. **Correct.**
   c. False. Dietary folic acid and vitamin B_{12} are required for erythrocyte synthesis.
   d. False. In adults, erythropoiesis takes place mainly in the ends of long bones.
   REF: Figure 4.5

10.
   a. **Correct.**
   b. False. MCH is the average amount of haemoglobin per erythrocyte.
   c. False. MCV is the volume of an average erythrocyte.
   d. False. Haematocrit (also called packed cell volume) is the volume of red cells in 1 L of blood.
   REF: Table 4.1

11.
   a. False. Erythropoietin is a hormone but acts on the red bone marrow to stimulate erythrocyte production.
   b. False. In erythropoietin deficiency, red blood cell numbers fall, which thins the blood.
   c. False. (See a.)
   d. **Correct.**
   REF: Page 66

12.
   a. False.
   b. False.
   c. **Correct.**
   d. False.
   REF: Figure 4.8

13.
  a. False.
  b. **Correct.**
  c. False.
  d. False.
  REF: Page 76
14.
  a. False. Megakaryoblasts give rise to platelets.
  b. False. Monoblasts give rise to monocytes.
  c. False. Lymphoblasts give rise to lymphocytes.
  d. **Correct.**
  REF: Figure 4.3
15.
  a. False.
  b. **Correct.**
  c. False.
  d. False.
  REF: Page 69
16.
  a. **Correct.**
  b. False.
  c. False.
  d. False.
  REF: Page 68
17.
  a. False.
  b. False.
  c. False.
  d. **Correct.**
  REF: Page 69
18.
  a. **Correct.**
  b. False.
  c. False.
  d. False.
  REF: Page 68
19.
  a. False. Kupffer cells are macrophages but are located in the liver.
  b. **Correct.**
  c. False. Macrophages are generally larger than other defence cells, and Kupffer cells are fixed in the liver.
  d. False. Macrophages are long-lived compared to other defence cells.
  REF: Figure 4.13
20.
  a. **Correct.** Ionising radiation is a risk factor, and genetic susceptibility is important in some cases.
  b. and c. True. As the cancerous white blood cell precursors multiply in the red bone marrow, they eliminate the precursor cells for erythrocytes and platelets, so there is anaemia and slow, impaired blood clotting.
  d. True.
  REF: Page 77

21.
   a. False.
   b. False.
   c. **Correct.**
   d. False.
   REF: Page 79

22.
   a. **Correct.**
   b. False.
   c. False.
   d. False.
   REF: Page 70

23.
   a. False. Erythrocytes, not platelets, are packed with haemoglobin.
   b. False. The average erythrocyte count is 4.5–6.5 million/mm^3 in adult males and 3.8–5.8 million/mm^3 in adult females; the average platelet count is 200,000–350,000/mm^3.
   c. False. Platelets are produced from megakaryoblasts, but erythrocytes are derived from erythroblasts.
   d. **Correct.**
   REF: Pages 63 and 70

24.
   a. False. Christmas factor is clotting factor IX.
   b. False. Calcium is clotting factor III.
   c. False. Stable factor is clotting factor VII.
   d. **Correct.**
   REF: Box 4.1

25.
   a. False. Thromboplastin, also called tissue factor, is clotting factor III and contributes to the external clotting pathway.
   b. **Correct.**
   c. False. Fibrin is the sticky, fibrous protein that forms the fundamental structure of a clot.
   d. False. Thrombin is the enzyme that releases fibrin from fibrinogen.
   REF: Page 71

26.
   a. **Correct.** Thromboplastin (tissue factor, or clotting factor III) contributes to the extrinsic pathway, which activates the final common pathway.
   b., c. and d. True. Prothrombin is converted to thrombin, which converts fibrinogen to fibrin.
   REF: Figure 4.15

27.
   a. False.
   b. **Correct.**
   c. False.
   d. False.
   REF: Page 65

28.
   a. **Correct.**
   b. False.
   c. False.
   d. False.
   REF: Page 79

29.
    a. False.
    b. **Correct.**
    c. False.
    d. False.
    REF: Page 72

30.
    a. False.
    b. False.
    c. **Correct.**
    d. False.
    REF: Page 75

CHAPTER 5

The Cardiovascular System

Feedback

1.
   a. False.
   b. False.
   c. **Correct.** Only veins have valves, to ensure one-way flow of blood.
   d. False.
   REF: Page 86

2.
   a. **Correct.**
   b. False.
   c. False.
   d. False.
   REF: Page 84

3.
   a. False. Their leaky walls allow liver cells to efficiently adjust the composition of blood. Bile is not secreted into the bloodstream.
   b. False. Blood flow through sinusoids is slow because of their large diameter.
   c. **Correct.**
   d. False. Liver cells receive their oxygen supply through branches of the hepatic artery, whereas the hepatic portal vein carries blood that has been through the gastrointestinal capillaries first, for cleaning and adjustment of its composition.
   REF: Page 83

4.
   a. False.
   b. **Correct.** Arterioles have smooth muscle in the middle layer of their walls, allowing rapid adjustment of their diameter, which controls the resistance to blood flow: when dilated, there is less resistance, and when constricted, resistance is higher.
   c. False.
   d. False.
   REF: Page 83

5.
   a. False. The capillary wall is a single layer of endothelial cells overlying a basement membrane.
   b. **Correct.**
   c. False. Plasma proteins can only cross the capillary wall when it is inflamed.
   d. False. The smallest capillaries are only 3–4 microns in diameter, which is even smaller than red blood cells (7 microns).
   REF: Page 83

6.
    a. **Correct.**
    b. False.
    c. False.
    d. False.
    REF: Page 85
7.
    a. False. Hydrostatic (blood) pressure falls from the arterial end of the capillary (about 5 kPa) to 2 kPa at the venous end because fluid has left the bloodstream through the leaky capillary walls.
    b. False. Although osmotic pressure pulls fluid into the blood, it opposes the hydrostatic (blood) pressure, which forces fluid into the tissues.
    c. False. Osmotic, not hydrostatic, pressure is due mainly to the presence of plasma proteins.
    d. **Correct.**
    REF: Figure 5.6
8.
    a. False. Lymph is the name given to tissue fluid once it enters the lymphatic system.
    b. **Correct.**
    c. and d. False. Both these terms refer to the fluid bathing cells.
    REF: Page 85
9.
    a., b. and c. False. All lie close to the apex of the heart.
    d. **Correct.**
    REF: Figure 5.7
10.
    a. False.
    b. False.
    c. **Correct.**
    d. False.
    REF: Figure 5.8
11.
    a. False. The myocardial cells are linked by intercalated discs but are branched.
    b. False. The intercalated discs between the myocardial cells allow direct cell-cell transmission of impulses from the sinoatrial node, so there is no need for every cell to have its own nerve supply.
    c. False. The conducting fibres are called Purkinje fibres.
    d. **Correct.**
    REF: Page 86
12.
    a. False. Pleural fluid is secreted by the visceral pleura and is the fluid in the pleural space surrounding the lungs.
    b. **Correct.**
    c. False. The endocardium lines the heart chambers.
    d. False. The fibrous pericardium is the outer protective layer.
    REF: Figure 5.9

13.

    a. **Correct.** The chordae tendinae fasten the cusps of the valves to the interior of the ventricles, so that during ventricular contraction, when pressure is rising, the valves snap shut without prolapsing back up into the atria.

    b. False. Valves are made of fibrous tissue, which does not conduct electricity.

    c. False. The right atrioventricular (AV) (tricuspid) valve has three cusps, but the left (mitral) AV valve is bicuspid (only has two cusps).

    d. False. The P wave represents atrial contraction, so the AV valves are open to allow blood to flow into the ventricles.

    REF: Figure 5.11

14.

    a. and b. False. These terms are sometimes used interchangeably, and both mean the inability of a damaged or fibrosed valve to close properly, allowing blood to leak backwards.

    c. **Correct.**

    d. False. Turbulent blood flow caused by incompetence results in abnormal heart sounds called murmurs that can be heard with a stethoscope.

    REF: Page 132

15.

    a. False.

    b. False.

    c. **Correct.**

    d. False.

    REF: Figure 5.16

16.

    a. False.

    b. False.

    c. **Correct.**

    d. False.

    REF: Page 89

17.

    a. False.

    b. **Correct.**

    c. False.

    d. False.

    REF: Page 90

18.

    a. **Correct.**

    b. False.

    c. False.

    d. False.

    REF: Page 134

19.

    a. False. The sinoatrial node sets the normal heart rate.

    b. False. The atrioventricular node is a backup pacemaker that keeps the heart beating in the event of sinoatrial node failure, but more slowly.

    c. False. The atrioventricular valves control blood flow between the atria and the ventricles.

    d. **Correct.**

    REF: Page 90

20.

    a. **Correct.** The heart spends about half of an average cardiac cycle (which lasts for about 0.8 sec) with both atria and ventricles relaxed.

    b. False. Ventricular contraction (systole) only lasts for 0.3 sec.

    c. False. Atrial systole only lasts for 0.1 sec.

    d. False. Atrial systole means atrial contraction.

    REF: Figure 5.17

21.

    a. False.

    b. False.

    c. **Correct.**

    d. False.

    REF: Page 93

22.

    a. False.

    b. **Correct.**

    c. False.

    d. False.

    REF: Page 92

23.

    a. False. The P wave shows atrial excitation.

    b. False. The T wave shows ventricular repolarisation.

    c. False. The P-R interval indicates the length of time taken for excitation to spread from the atria to the ventricles.

    d. **Correct.**

    REF: Page 94

24.

    a. False.

    b. False.

    c. **Correct.**

    d. False.

    REF: Page 135

25.

    a. **Correct.** This is the peak pressure in the system, generated by the powerful contraction of the left ventricle.

    b. False. The diastolic pressure is recorded when the ventricles are relaxed and the pressure in the system is at its lowest.

    c. False. Pulse pressure is the difference between systolic and diastolic pressures.

    d. False. The mean arterial pressure is the average arterial pressure over one cardiac cycle.

    REF: Page 96

26.

    a. False. The atria are filling, and because the ventricles are nearly empty, pressure is higher in the atria than the ventricles, pushing the atrioventricular (AV) valves open.

    b. **Correct.**

    c. False. Constant return of blood into the atria is increasing pressure in these chambers, but the ventricular pressure is low because the ventricles are nearly empty.

    d. False. The atria are continually receiving blood from the venae cavae, this increased pressure pushes the AV valves open, and blood flows passively into the ventricles. In the healthy heart, most ventricular filling occurs this way, and atrial contraction merely tops it up.

    REF: Figure 5.17

27.
   a. **Correct.**
   b. and c. False. The end-diastolic volume is the volume of blood in the ventricle immediately before contraction, but not all this blood is ejected as the stroke volume; typically, about 70% is pumped out, leaving about 30% in the ventricle.
   d. False. Systolic pressure minus diastolic pressure is the pulse pressure.
   REF: Page 94

28.
   a. False: the smooth muscle of the blood vessel wall is in the tunica media.
   b. **Correct.**
   c. False. The cardiovascular centre is in the medulla oblongata in the brainstem.
   d. False. Relaxation of vascular smooth muscle decreases peripheral resistance.
   REF: Page 96

29.
   a. False.
   b. **Correct.**
   c. False.
   d. False.
   REF: Figure 5.22

30.
   a. False.
   b. False.
   c. **Correct.** Because the left ventricle pumps blood into the systemic circulation, a sustained rise in blood pressure greatly increases its workload.
   d. False.
   REF: Page 137

31.
   a. False. Adrenaline is a sympathetic hormone.
   b. and c. False. The heart has both sympathetic and parasympathetic nerve supply, the most important determinants of heart rate.
   d. **Correct.**
   REF: Page 95

32.
   a. **Correct.** Liver failure reduces plasma protein levels, reducing the osmotic pressure of the blood and allowing fluid to escape from the bloodstream and accumulate in the peritoneal cavity.
   b. False. Lymphatic obstruction in the peritoneum can prevent drainage from the abdominal cavity, but if the axillary drainage is blocked, it will cause oedema of the arm.
   c. False. Hypotension reduces hydrostatic pressure and would oppose the movement of fluid into the tissues.
   d. False. Elevated plasma protein levels increases the osmotic pressure of the blood and would pull fluid into the bloodstream from the tissues to reduce it.
   REF: Page 130

33.
   a. False. The pulmonary circulation contains only about 10% of the body's blood.
   b. False. Blood carried to the lungs by the pulmonary artery is deoxygenated.
   c. False. The right ventricle pumps blood to the lungs (through the pulmonary artery).
   d. **Correct.** The average pressure in the pulmonary circulation is only 15 mmHg because higher pressures force fluid out of the bloodstream and into the alveoli.
   REF: Page 101

34.
 a. False.
 b. **Correct.**
 c. False.
 d. False.
 REF: Figure 5.25

35.
 a. False.
 b. False.
 c. **Correct.**
 d. False.
 REF: Figure 5.26

36.
 a. False.
 b. False.
 c. False.
 d. **Correct.**
 REF: Figure 5.24

37.
 a. False. It is a complete circular channel but lies on the underside of the brain in the subarachnoid space.
 b. **Correct.**
 c. False. The internal carotids contribute, but not the temporal artery, which supplies the scalp.
 d. False. Branches of the circulus arteriosus supply most of the brain.
 REF: Figure 5.31

38.
 a. **Correct.**
 b. False.
 c. False.
 d. False.
 REF: Figure 5.33

39.
 a. False.
 b. False.
 c. **Correct.** All the others are present as paired (right and left) arteries
 d. False.
 REF: Figure 5.37

40.
 a. False.
 b. False.
 c. **Correct.**
 d. False.
 REF: Figure 5.38

41.
 a. False.
 b. False.
 c. False.
 d. **Correct.**
 REF: Figure 5.41

42.

b. **Correct.**

a., c. and d. False. All of these are associated with both conditions, although the stiffening of arterial walls is due to calcified fatty plaques in atherosclerosis and to the laying down of calcified fibrous tissue in arteriosclerosis.

REF: Pages 125 and 126

43.

a. False. The placenta is an interface, but there is no direct contact between maternal and fetal blood.

b. **Correct.**

c. False. The placenta is operational in the second and third trimesters of pregnancy.

d. False. The placenta protects against many, but not all, infections and toxins.

REF: Page 116

44.

a. **Correct.**

b. False. The ductus venosus bypasses the fetal liver.

c. False. The foramen ovale shunts blood from the right atrium to the left atrium.

d. False. Although the fetal intestines are not in use, there is no specific bypass mechanism shunting blood away from them.

REF: Page 119

45.

a. **Correct.**

b. False.

c. False.

d. False.

REF: Figure 5.28

46.

a. False. The aorta has little or no smooth muscle in its walls, to prevent constriction of the artery, which would increase the force required from the left ventricle to pump blood through it.

b. and c. False. Both fibrous tissue and the endothelial lining are present in all arteries.

d. **Correct.** The aorta has to expand readily to accept the blood pumped from the left ventricle, to minimise the workload of the left ventricle. The elastic tissue expands and then recoils, helping to push the blood forward into distal arteries.

REF: Page 83

47.

a. False. The fibrous skeleton becomes stiffer, increasing the workload of the myocardium.

b. **Correct.**

c. False. The ageing healthy heart responds less well to adrenaline and noradrenaline than the younger heart.

d. False. Regular exercise has strongly beneficial effects on the heart throughout the lifespan.

REF: Page 120

48.

a. False. The openings to the pulmonary arteries are stenosed, increasing the workload of the right ventricle (which is why this chamber is usually hypertrophic).

b. False. There is usually a ventricular septal defect, which is an abnormal hole between the two ventricles.

c. False. The origin of the aorta is displaced to the right.

d. **Correct.**

REF: Page 135

49.
   a. False.
   b. **Correct.**
   c. False.
   d. False.
   REF: Page 128
50.
   a. False.
   b. False.
   c. **Correct.**
   d. False.
   REF: Figure 5.38

CHAPTER 6

The Lymphatic System

Feedback

1.
    a. False.
    b. **Correct.**
    c. False.
    d. False.
    REF: Figure 6.1

2.
    a. False.
    b. False.
    c. **Correct.**
    d. False.
    REF: Figure 6.1

3.
    a. **Correct.** The thoracic duct drains the lower parts of the body, including the gastrointestinal tract, as well as the left arm, shoulder and left side of the head and neck.
    b. False. The right lymphatic duct drains the right arm and shoulder and the right side of the head, neck and thorax.
    c. False. The cisternae chyli is the dilated section at the origin of the thoracic duct.
    d. False. The subclavian duct is not a biological structure.
    REF: Page 143

4.
    a. False. Although lymph and plasma are very similar in composition, they are not identical.
    b. False. Plasma contains more protein than lymph.
    c. False. Lymph contains numerous white blood cells.
    d. **Correct.** Lymph drains away large particulate matter from tissues, including bacteria and debris from damaged cells.
    REF: Page 143

5.
    a. **Correct.** In addition to this 'lymphatic pump', lymphatic vessels also have one-way valves, and compression of lymphatic vessels by adjacent skeletal muscles squeezes lymph forward.
    b. False. The heart does not pump lymph.
    c. False. There are no cilia in lymphatic vessels.
    d. False. Although gravity helps (e.g., lying down or elevating the feet improves tissue drainage), lymphatic drainage continues efficiently even against gravity because of the measures described in a. (above).
    REF: Page 143

6.

    a. False. The middle layer contains smooth muscle; the term 'skeletal muscle pump' refers to the squeezing of lymphatic vessels by adjacent skeletal muscles.

    b. **Correct.** A fibrous covering, a middle layer of elastic tissue and smooth muscle and a single cell–thick lining, the endothelium.

    c. False. The elastic tissue is found in the middle layer.

    d. False. The endothelium lines the vessel.

    REF: Page 143

7.

    a. False.

    b. False.

    c. **Correct.**

    d. False.

    REF: Page 144

8.

    a. False. Lymph nodes filter and clean lymph but not blood.

    b. False. The internal partitions are formed from extensions of the outer capsule and are called trabeculae.

    c. False. A lymph node is usually supplied with four or five afferent vessels bringing lymph in, although there is only one efferent vessel carrying it away.

    d. **Correct.**

    REF: Page 144

9.

    a. False.

    b. False.

    c. False.

    d. **Correct.** Mastectomy is removal of all or part of the breast, and the local lymph nodes draining the breast (and therefore in which malignant cells may have become established) are the axillary group of lymph nodes.

    REF: Figure 6.1

10.

    a. False.

    b. **Correct.**

    c. False.

    d. False.

    REF: Figure 6.1

11.

    a. False.

    b. False.

    c. **Correct.**

    d. False.

    REF: Page 144

12.

    a. False. Lymphadenitis is infection of lymph nodes.

    b. **Correct.**

    c. False. Lymphangitis is inflammation of lymph vessels.

    d. False. Lymphoedema is tissue swelling due to blocked lymph drainage.

    REF: Page 150, Table 6.1

13.
   a. False. Non-Hodgkin lymphoma is more common than Hodgkin lymphoma.
   b. False. This is a feature of Hodgkin lymphoma.
   c. **Correct.** This also applies to Hodgkin lymphoma.
   d. False. Bone marrow involvement is common.
   REF: Page 150

14.
   a. **Correct.**
   b. False.
   c. False.
   d. False.
   REF: Page 145

15.
   a. False.
   b. **Correct.**
   c. False.
   d. False.
   REF: Page 146

16.
   a. False. The spleen lies immediately below the diaphragm.
   b. False. The spleen stores blood, but not lymph.
   c. False. The spleen can only store about 350 mL of blood.
   d. **Correct.** Additionally, in times of great need, the spleen may produce red blood cells in adults too.
   REF: Page 146

17.
   a. False.
   b. **Correct.**
   c. False.
   d. False.
   REF: Page 147

18.
   a. **Correct.** The T in T-lymphocytes (T-cells) stands for thymus, indicating the key role this gland plays in the production of mature T-cells.
   b. False.
   c. False.
   d. False.
   REF: Page 147

19.
   a. False. Thymosin is produced by the thymus gland.
   b False. The thymus gland begins to regress at puberty, so thymosin levels decline from this time too.
   c. **Correct.**
   d. False. Thymosin is produced by epithelial tissues of the thymus gland.
   REF: Page 147

20.
   a. **Correct.** Enlargement of the thymus is also sometimes found in other autoimmune disorders such as myasthenia gravis.
   b. False.
   c. False.
   d. False.
   REF: Page 151 ·

CHAPTER 7

The Nervous System

Feedback

1.
    a. False. Neurones have only one axon.
    b. False. Neurones have many dendrites.
    c. False. Neurones are not capable of dividing.
    d. **Correct.** Neurones can only synthesise chemical energy (ATP) from glucose.
    REF: Page 155

2.
    a. **Correct.** The cell membrane is polarised in the resting state.
    b. False. Potassium (K^+) is the principal intracellular cation.
    c. False. At rest, K^+ tends to diffuse into the cells.
    d. False. Depolarisation occurs when Na^+ floods into the cells.
    REF: Pages 156 and 157

3.
    a. False. Nerve impulses can only travel way along a neurone, from the cell body to the axon terminals.
    b. False. Nerve impulses travel more quickly in myelinated neurones.
    c. **Correct.** Nerve impulses travel by saltatory conduction in myelinated neurones.
    d. False. Nerve impulses cannot travel during the refractory period.
    REF: Page 157 and Figure 7.5

4.
    a. False. The presynaptic neurone has many synaptic knobs.
    b. False. Neurotransmitters are stored in vesicles within the synaptic knobs.
    c. **Correct.** Neurotransmitters diffuse across the synaptic cleft and can only act on specific receptor sites.
    d. False. Neurotransmitters usually have an excitatory effect on the postsynaptic membrane, but some have an inhibitory effect.
    REF: Page 157

5.
    a. **Correct.** Epineurium is the fibrous tissue that encloses bundles of nerve fibres.
    b. False. Endoneurium is the delicate tissue that surrounds each individual nerve fibre.
    c. False. Perineurium is the smooth connective tissue that surrounds several bundles of nerve fibres.
    d. False. Myelin is contained within Schwann cells, which wrap around the axons of myelinated neurones.
    REF: Page 158, Figure 7.9

6.
  a. False. Motor nerves are also known as efferent nerves.
  b. False. Motor nerves carry impulses from the central nervous system to effector organs (muscles and glands).
  c. False. Sensory nerves include those with endings in the baroreceptors.
  d. **Correct.** When involved in skeletal muscle contraction (voluntary or reflex), motor nerves are also known as somatic nerves.
  REF: Pages 158 and 159

7.
  a. **Correct.** Oligodendrocytes are the glial cells that form and maintain myelin in the central nervous system.
  b. False. Astrocytes are the main supporting tissue in the central nervous system. Some have processes that form the blood-brain barrier.
  c. False. Microglia migrate into the nervous system before birth, and inflammation there causes them to enlarge, become phagocytic and migrate to affected areas of the central nervous system.
  d. False. Ependymal cells line the ventricles of the brain.
  REF: Page 160 and Figure 7.12

8.
  a. False.
  b. **Correct.** Some astrocytes have foot processes that form the blood-brain barrier.
  c. False.
  d. False.
  REF: Page 160

9.
  a. **Correct.** The dura mater is the outermost of the meninges.
  b. False. The arachnoid mater lies between the dura mater and the pia mater.
  c. False. The pia mater lies innermost.
  d. False. The subarachnoid space separates the arachnoid and pia maters, and contains cerebrospinal fluid.
  REF: Page 162, Figure 7.14

10.
  a. **Correct.** The falx cerebri is formed by the inner layer of the dura mater where it sweeps inwards between the cerebral hemispheres.
  b. False. The falx cerebelli is formed where the inner layer of the dura mater sweeps inwards between the cerebellar hemispheres.
  c. False. The tentorium cerebelli is formed by the inner layer of the dura mater where it sweeps inwards between the cerebrum and cerebellum.
  d. False.
  REF: Page 162, Figure 7.14A

11.
  a. False.
  b. False.
  c. **Correct.** Spinal dura mater forms a loose sheath around the spinal cord, extending from the foramen magnum to the 2nd sacral vertebra.
  d. False.
  REF: Page 162, Figure 7.14A

12.
  a. False.
  b. **Correct.** Diagnostic dyes, local anaesthetics and analgesics are injected into the epidural space.
  c. False.
  d. False.
  REF: Page 162

13.
  a. False.
  b. False.
  c. **Correct.** Beyond the end of the cord, the pia mater continues as the filum terminale.
  d. False.
  REF: Page 162

14.
  a. False. The outermost dura mater consists of two layers of dense fibrous tissue, neither of which dip into the fissures.
  b. False. The arachnoid mater accompanies the inner layer of dura mater and passes over the convolutions of the brain.
  c. **Correct.** The pia mater adheres to the brain, completely covering the convolutions and dipping into each fissure.
  d. False.
  REF: Page 162, Figure 7.14A

15.
  a. False. The right and left lateral ventricles are not connected to each other.
  b. False. The lateral ventricles are linked to the third ventricle via the interventricular foramina.
  c. **Correct.** The third ventricle is connected to the fourth ventricle by the cerebral aqueduct.
  d. False. The fourth ventricle is continuous with the central canal of spinal cord below.
  REF: Page 163, Figure 7.15

16.
  a. False. The lateral ventricles lie within the cerebral hemispheres, one on each side of the median plane.
  b. False. The third ventricle is situated between the two parts of the thalamus.
  c. **Correct.** The fourth ventricle lies between the cerebellum and the pons.
  d. False.
  REF: Page 163, Figure 7.14A

17.
  a. False. CSF is secreted at the rate of 1.5 mL/min.
  b. **Correct.** CSF is slightly alkaline.
  c. False. CSF has a specific gravity of 1.005.
  d. False. Leukocytes are not a normal constituent of CSF.
  REF: Pages 163–164

18.
  a. **Correct.**
  b. False. Cerebral oedema is the accumulation of fluid in the interstitial spaces or cells in the brain.
  c. False. Papilloedema is oedema around the optic disc.
  d. False. Herniation is displacement of the brain from its usual compartment.
  REF: Page 193

19.
   a. False.
   b. False.
   c. **Correct.** The pons is a part of the brain stem.
   d. False.
   REF: Page 165, Figure 7.17
20.
   a. False.
   b. False.
   c. **Correct.** The approximate volume of blood supplied to the brain is 750 mL/min.
   d. False.
   REF: Page 165
21.
   a. False. The cerebrum is divided by a deep cleft, the longitudinal cerebral fissure, into the right and left cerebral hemispheres.
   b. False. The cerebrum occupies the anterior and middle cranial fossae.
   c. **Correct.** The cerebrum consists of gyri (convolutions) separated by sulci (fissures).
   d. False. The superficial part of the cerebrum is composed of grey matter, forming the cerebral cortex, and the deeper layers consist of nerve fibres (white matter).
   REF: Page 165
22.
   a. **Correct.** Association fibres connect different parts of the same cerebral hemisphere by extending from one gyrus to another.
   b. False. Commissural fibres connect corresponding areas of the two cerebral hemispheres.
   c. False. Projection fibres connect the cerebral cortex with grey matter of lower parts of the brain and with the spinal cord.
   d. False. The pyramidal (corticospinal) tracts are the motor fibres within the internal capsule.
   REF: Page 165
23.
   a. False.
   b. **Correct.** The corpus callosum is the largest and most important commissural tract.
   c. False.
   d. False.
   REF: Page 165
24.
   a. **Correct.**
   b. False. The areas representing the different parts of the body are proportionately related to the complexity of their movement, not their size.
   c. False.
   d. False. Motor control is contralateral (opposite side), not ipsilateral (same side) i.e., the motor area of the right hemisphere controls voluntary muscle movement on the left side of the body and vice versa.
   REF: Page 167
25.
   a. False. The primary motor area lies in the frontal lobe, immediately anterior to the central sulcus.
   b. **Correct.** Broca's (motor speech) area is situated in the frontal lobe, just superior to the lateral sulcus.
   c. False. The somatosensory area lies immediately posterior to the central sulcus.
   d. False. The visual area lies posterior to the parieto-occipital sulcus.
   REF: Page 167, Figure 7.20

26.
    a. False.
    b. False.
    c. False.
    d. **Correct.** Wernicke's area is the sensory speech area.
    REF: Page 168

27.
    a. False.
    b. False.
    c. **Correct.** The vital centres lie in the medulla oblongata.
    d. False.
    REF: Page 170

28.
    a. False. Around 50% of brain tumours are secondary tumours.
    b. False. Brain tumours usually arise from glial cells because nerve cells cannot normally divide.
    c. False. Astrocytomas and medulloblastomas are the cause of most brain tumours in children.
    d. **Correct.** Brain tumours are described as benign when they are slow growing.
    REF: Page 203

29.
    a. False.
    b. **Correct.** The cerebellum enables coordination of posture, balance and equilibrium.
    c. False.
    d. False.
    REF: Page 171

30.
    a. False.
    b. False.
    c. **Correct.**
    d. False.
    REF: Page 195, Figure 7.48

31.
    a. False.
    b. **Correct.**
    c. False.
    d. False.
    REF: Page 198

32.
    a. False.
    b. False.
    c. False.
    d. **Correct.**
    REF: Page 196

33.
    a. **Correct.** The spinal cord has an anterior shallow median fissure and a posterior deep posterior median septum.
    b. False. Grey matter in the centre is surrounded by white matter.
    c. False. The spinal cord is about 45 cm long in adult males.
    d. False. Arrangement of the grey matter resembles the shape of the letter H.
    REF: Page 173

34.
  a. False.
  b. False.
  c. False. Neurone 2 of all these sensory nerves decussates upon entering the spinal cord.
  d. **Correct.** Proprioceptor fibres going to the cerebellum do not decussate.
  REF: Page 174, Table 7.1

35.
  a. False.
  b. **Correct.** The cell bodies of lower motor neurones are located in anterior horn of grey matter in the spinal cord.
  c. False.
  d. False.
  REF: Page 174

36.
  a. **Correct.**
  b. False.
  c. False.
  d. False.
  REF: Page 199

37.
  a. False.
  b. False.
  c. **Correct.** The pupillary light reflex is an autonomic reflex.
  d. False.
  REF: Page 176

38.
  a. **Correct.** The smallest plexus is the coccygeal plexus.
  b. False.
  c. False.
  d. False.
  REF: Page 182

39.
  a. False.
  b. **Correct.** The phrenic nerve originates from cervical nerve roots 3, 4 and 5.
  c. False.
  d. False.
  REF: Page 178

40.
  a. False.
  b. False.
  c. False.
  d. **Correct.** The radial nerve is the largest branch of brachial plexus.
  REF: Page 179

41.
  a. False.
  b. False.
  c. False.
  d. **Correct.** The sciatic nerve, which is a branch of sacral plexus, is the largest nerve in the body.
  REF: Page 181

42.
    a. False.
    b. False.
    c. **Correct.** The external anal sphincter is supplied by the perineal branch of pudendal nerve.
    d. False.
    REF: Page 182

43.
    a. **Correct.** The vagus nerve has the most extensive distribution, supplying the smooth muscle and secretory glands of many organs, including those of the respiratory, urinary and digestive tracts.
    b. False.
    c. False.
    d. False.
    REF: Page 185, Figure 7.43

44.
    a. **Correct.** The trochlear nerve is a motor nerve supplying the superior oblique muscles of the eyes. It is not a branch of the trigeminal nerve.
    b. False.
    c. False.
    d. False. The trigeminal nerve has three branches: the ophthalmic, maxillary and mandibular nerves.
    REF: Page 185, Figure 7.42

45.
    a. **Correct.** The glossopharyngeal nerve is essential for the swallowing and gag reflexes.
    b. False.
    c. False.
    d. False.
    REF: Page 185

46.
    a., c. and d. True. The facial, glossopharyngeal and vagus nerves are mixed nerves.
    b. **Correct.** The vestibulocochlear (auditory) nerves are sensory nerves.
    REF: Page 185

47.
    a. False. It is a thoracolumbar outflow.
    b. False. There are three prevertebral sympathetic ganglia in the abdominal cavity.
    c. False.
    d. **Correct.** Sympathetic cholinergic nerves form the postganglionic neurones to the skin, sweat glands and skeletal muscles.
    REF: Pages 186 and 187, Figure 7.44

48.
    a. False.
    b. **Correct.** The parasympathetic nervous system always uses acetylcholine as its neurotransmitter.
    c. False.
    d. False.
    REF: Page 188, Figures 7.8 and 7.45

49.

    a. True.

    b. True.

    c. **Correct.** Increased motility and secretion in the stomach and small intestine is an effect of parasympathetic stimulation.

    d. True.

    REF: Page 189

50.

    a. False. Referred pain from the heart is felt in the left shoulder.

    b. False. Referred pain from the uterus is felt in the lower back.

    c. False. Appendicular pain is visceral (not referred) pain.

    d. **Correct.** Referred pain from the kidney and ureter is felt in the loin and groin.

    REF: Page 190 and Table 7.3

CHAPTER 8

The Special Senses

Feedback

1.
   a. False. The external acoustic meatus is S-shaped and about 2.5 cm long.
   b. False. The external acoustic meatus carries sound waves to the middle ear.
   c. **Correct.** The external acoustic meatus is lined with skin containing ceruminous glands, which are modified sweat glands.
   d. False. It is the pharyngotympanic tube that is normally closed but, when there is unequal pressure across the tympanic membrane, e.g., at high altitude, can be opened by swallowing or yawning, and the ears 'pop', equalising the pressure again.
   REF: Pages 208 and 209

2.
   a. False.
   b. False.
   c. **Correct.** The tympanic cavity is largely bounded by the temporal bone.
   d. False.
   REF: Page 209

3.
   a. False.
   b. **Correct.** The incus is the middle anvil-shaped bone that possesses long and short processes.
   c. False.
   d. False.
   REF: Page 209, Figure 8.3

4.
   a. False.
   b. False.
   c. False. The vestibule, semicircular canals and cochlea are all parts of the inner ear.
   d. **Correct.** The pharyngotympanic tube links the middle ear to the throat.
   REF: Page 210

5.
   a. **Correct.** The membranous labyrinth lies within the bony labyrinth.
   b. False. The bony labyrinth is filled with perilymph.
   c. False. The auditory receptors are dendrites of specialised afferent nerve endings.
   d. False. The cochlear duct contains endolymph.
   REF: Page 210

6.
  a. False.
  b. False.
  c. False.
  d. **Correct.** The auditory area in the temporal lobe of the cerebrum perceives sound.
  REF: Pages 211 and 212

7.
  a., c. and d. False. Ototoxic drugs, long-term exposure to excessive noise and Ménière's disease cause sensorineural hearing loss.
  b. **Correct.**
  REF: Box 8.1

8.
  a. **Correct.** The utricle contains hair cells for balance.
  b. False.
  c. False.
  d. False. Hair cells for balance are not found in the semicircular canals, the spiral organ or the basilar membrane.
  REF: Page 212

9.
  a. False.
  b. False.
  c. **Correct.** The uveal tract is the middle layer of the eyeball wall.
  d. False.
  REF: Page 214

10.
  a. **Correct.** The choroid lines the posterior five-sixths of the sclera.
  b. False. The choroid has an abundant supply of blood vessels.
  c. False. The sclera gives attachment to the extrinsic muscles of the eye.
  d. False.
  REF: Page 214

11.
  a. True. The lens is attached to the ciliary body by radiating suspensory ligaments that resemble the spokes of a wheel.
  b. True. Many of the smooth muscle fibres are circular, so the ciliary muscle constricts rather than dilates the pupil.
  c. **Correct.** The epithelial cells secrete aqueous fluid into the anterior chamber of the eye.
  d. True. The ciliary body is supplied by parasympathetic branches of the oculomotor (third) cranial nerve.
  REF: Page 214

12.
  a. False. The cornea is a transparent epithelial membrane.
  b. False. The choroid is chocolate brown and does not determine the colour of the eye, as it lines the posterior aspect of the sclera.
  c. **Correct.** The pigment cells in the iris determine eye colour.
  d. False. The retina is composed of several layers of nerve cell bodies and their axons, and does not determine eye colour.
  REF: Page 214

13.

    a. False.

    b. False.

    c. False.

    d. **Correct.** Cataracts cause opacity of the lens.

    REF: Page 225, Figure 8.26

14.

    a. **Correct.** The fovea centralis is a little depression in the centre of the macula lutea (yellow spot).

    b. False. The optic disc (blind spot) is situated 0.5 cm to the nasal side of the macula lutea.

    c. False. The ciliary body is the anterior continuation of choroid, consisting of ciliary muscle and secretory epithelial cells.

    d. False. The iris is the visible coloured ring at the front of the eye.

    REF: Page 215, Figure 8.11

15.

    a. False.

    b. **Correct.** The central retinal artery and vein are encased in the optic nerve, which enters the eye at the optic disc.

    c. False.

    d. False.

    REF: Page 215

16.

    a. True.

    b. True.

    c. True.

    d. **Correct.** The lens, lens capsule and cornea do not have a blood supply.

    REF: Page 216

17.

    a. False.

    b. **Correct.** The normal intraocular pressure remains fairly constant at 10–20 mmHg.

    c. False.

    d. False.

    REF: Page 216

18.

    a. False.

    b. False.

    c. False.

    d. **Correct.**

    REF: Page 228

19.

    a. **Correct.** The optic tracts contain nasal fibres from one eye and temporal fibres from the other eye.

    b. False.

    c. False.

    d. False.

    REF: Page 216, Figure 8.13

20.
   a. False.
   b. **Correct.** The optic radiations terminate in the visual area of the cerebral cortex in the occipital lobes of the cerebrum.
   c. False.
   d. False.
   REF: Page 216, Figure 8.13

21.
   a. True.
   b. True.
   c. True.
   d. **Correct.** All of the above processes are involved in producing a clear visual image of nearby objects.
   REF: Page 218

22.
   a. **Correct.** Microwaves have a longer wavelength than violet light rays, X-rays and gamma rays.
   b. False.
   c. False.
   d. False.
   REF: Page 217, Figure 8.15

23.
   a. False. Rods are sensitive to light.
   b. **Correct.** Cones are sensitive to colour and light.
   c. False. Rhodopsin is the light-sensitive pigment present only in rods.
   d. False.
   REF: Pages 219 and 220

24.
   a. False. Colour blindness is a condition in which affected individuals see colours but cannot always differentiate between them.
   b. False. Dark adaptation is a temporary visual impairment when moving from an area of bright light to dark area, and is due to degeneration of rhodopsin in bright light.
   c. False. Binocular vision provides an accurate assessment of the distance, depth, height and width of objects.
   d. **Correct.** People with monocular vision find it difficult to judge the speed and distance of an approaching vehicle.
   REF: Page 220

25.
   a. False. The oculomotor nerve (third cranial nerve) supplies the medial rectus muscle of the eye.
   b. False. The trochlear nerve (fourth cranial nerve) supplies the superior oblique muscle of the eye.
   c. **Correct.** The abducent nerve (sixth cranial nerve) supplies the lateral rectus muscle of the eye.
   d. False. The oculomotor nerve (third cranial nerve) supplies the intrinsic eye muscles of the iris and ciliary body.
   REF: Page 221, Table 8.1

26.
    a. False. The superior rectus muscle rotates the eyeball upward.
    b. False. The inferior rectus muscle rotates the eyeball downward.
    c. False. The superior oblique muscle rotates the eyeball downward and outward.
    d. **Correct.** The inferior oblique muscle rotates the eyeball upward and outward.
    REF: Page 221, Table 8.1
27.
    a. False.
    b. **Correct.** Tarsal glands are modified sebaceous glands found in eyelid margins.
    c. False.
    d. False.
    REF: Page 222, Figure 8.22
28.
    a. True. The glossopharyngeal nerve (seventh cranial nerve) carries the sense of taste.
    b. True. The facial nerve (ninth cranial nerve) carries the sense of taste.
    c. True. The vagus nerve (tenth cranial nerve) carries the sense of taste.
    d. **Correct.** The olfactory nerve (first cranial nerve) carries the sense of smell.
    REF: Page 224
29.
    a. **Correct.** The taste area is located in the parietal lobe of the cerebral cortex.
    b. False.
    c. False.
    d. False.
    REF: Page 224
30.
    a. False.
    b. **Correct.**
    c. False.
    d. False.
    REF: Page 225

CHAPTER 9

The Endocrine System

Feedback

1.
  a. **Correct.**
  b. False.
  c. False.
  d. False. The pineal, pituitary and parathyroid glands have primary endocrine functions.
  REF: Page 234, Figure 9.1

2.
  a., b. and d. False. Cortisone, thyroxine and aldosterone are lipid-based hormones.
  c. **Correct.** Insulin is a peptide hormone.
  REF: Page 235, Box 9.1

3.
  a. False.
  b. False.
  c. **Correct.** Release of oxytocin is regulated by a positive feedback mechanism.
  d. False. Secretion of LH, thyroxine and glucagon is regulated by negative feedback mechanisms.
  REF: Pages 238 and 239

4.
  a. False.
  b. **Correct.** The pituitary gland weighs about 500 mg.
  c. False.
  d. False.
  REF: Page 235

5.
  a. False.
  b. **Correct.** The pituitary gland is supplied by branches of the internal carotid artery.
  c. False.
  d. False.
  REF: Page 235

6.
  a. False.
  b. **Correct.** The posterior pituitary is formed from nervous tissue and consists of nerve cells surrounded by supporting cells called pituicytes.
  c. False.
  d. False.
  REF: Page 238, Figure 9.3B

7.

a. False. The pituitary portal system carries blood from the hypothalamus to the anterior lobe.

b. False. Releasing hormones are produced by the hypothalamus.

c. False. Trophic hormones are produced by the anterior lobe.

d. **Correct.** Oxytocin is released by axon terminals within the posterior lobe.

REF: Page 236, Figure 9.3

8.

a. False. Acromegaly affects adults; gigantism occurs in children.

b. False. Acromegaly is associated with hypersecretion of growth hormone (GH).

c. **Correct.** Acromegaly causes excessive growth of the hands and feet.

d. False. Acromegaly is usually caused by a hormone-secreting tumour of the anterior pituitary.

REF: Page 249, Figure 9.16

9.

a. **Correct.** GH is the most abundant hormone synthesised by the anterior pituitary.

b. False.

c. False.

d. False.

REF: Page 236

10.

a. False. GH stimulates growth and division of most body cells and, although secretion rises during deep sleep, it is not associated with the sleep pattern.

b. False. Thyroid hormones are essential for normal growth and development.

c. False. Prolactin maintains lactation.

d. **Correct.** ACTH maintains circadian rhythms and is associated with the sleep pattern and adjustment to changes in time zone, i.e., jet lag.

REF: Pages 236–238

11.

a. False. Secretion of GH is greater at night during sleep.

b. False. Release of TSH is lowest in the early evening and highest during night.

c. **Correct.** ACTH levels are highest at 8 a.m. and fall to their lowest about midnight.

d. False. No such effect is described for ADH.

REF: Page 238

12.

a. True. LH stimulates interstitial cells of the testis in males to secrete testosterone and is involved in the secretion of oestrogen and progesterone in females during the menstrual cycle.

b. True. FSH stimulates production of gametes by the gonads in both sexes and is also involved in secretion of oestrogen and progesterone in females during the menstrual cycle.

c. **Correct.** LH and FSH are both sex hormones secreted by the anterior pituitary.

d. False.

REF: Page 238

13.

a. True. Oxytocin stimulates more forceful uterine contractions and greater stretching of the uterine cervix.

b. True. Oxytocin causes contraction of the myoepithelial cells of the milk ducts, leading to milk ejection.

c. True. Oxytocin increases smooth muscle contraction during sexual arousal.

d. **Correct.** Oxytocin acts in all three ways described above.

REF: Pages 238 and 239

14.
    a. False.
    b. **Correct.** ADH secretion will be reduced due to a fall in the osmotic pressure of the blood following a large fluid intake. Less water will be reabsorbed, and more urine will be produced.
    c. False.
    d. False.
    REF: Page 239

15.
    a. True. ADH acts on distal convoluted tubules by increasing their permeability to water and more glomerular filtrate is reabsorbed.
    b. **Correct.** ADH does not act on proximal convoluted tubules.
    c. True. ADH acts on collecting ducts by increasing their permeability to water and more glomerular filtrate is reabsorbed.
    d. True. ADH causes smooth muscle contraction of small arteries, leading to vasoconstriction.
    REF: Pages 239 and 240

16.
    a. **Correct.** The approximate weight of the thyroid gland is 25 g.
    b. False.
    c. False.
    d. False.
    REF: Page 240

17.
    a. False.
    b. False.
    c. **Correct.** Tetany is a sign of hypoparathyroidism.
    d. False.
    REF: Page 252, Figure 9.19

18.
    a. **Correct.** Secretion of T3 and T4 begins in the third month of fetal life and is increased at puberty and in women during the reproductive years, especially during pregnancy.
    b. False.
    c. False.
    d. False.
    REF: Page 241

19.
    a. **Correct.** Weight gain is a common effect of hypothyroidism.
    b. False.
    c. False.
    d. False. Anxiety, hair loss and heat intolerance are common symptoms of hyperthyroidism.
    REF: Page 241, Table 9.3

20.
    a. False. Exophthalmos is a sign of hyperthyroidism.
    b. False.
    c. **Correct.** Simple goitre is swelling of the thyroid gland; it is a form of hypothyroidism.
    d. False.
    REF: Page 251, Figure 9.17

21.
  a. False. Calcitonin is secreted by the parafollicular or C-cells in the thyroid gland.
  b. **Correct.** Calcitonin acts on bone cells and promotes storage of calcium.
  c. False. Calcitonin lowers raised blood calcium levels.
  d. False. Calcitonin inhibits reabsorption of calcium by the renal tubules.
  REF: Page 241

22.
  a. False. Aldosterone is a mineralocorticoid hormone.
  b. **Correct.** Corticosterone is a glucocorticoid produced in small amounts by the adrenal cortex.
  c. False. Testosterone is an androgen (male sex hormone).
  d. False.
  REF: Page 243

23.
  a. True. Glucocorticoids increase plasma glucose levels by stimulating breakdown of glycogen and gluconeogenesis.
  b. True. Glucocorticoids stimulate lipolysis, raising plasma levels of free fatty acids.
  c. **Correct.** Calcitonin maintains blood calcium levels by lowering raised blood calcium levels.
  d. True. Glucocorticoids stimulate breakdown of proteins, increasing amino acid levels in the plasma.
  REF: Pages 243 and 244

24.
  a. True. Juxtaglomerular cells of the kidney secrete the enzyme renin when renal blood flow is reduced or blood sodium levels fall.
  b. True. The liver synthesises the enzyme precursor angiotensinogen (converted to angiotensin 1 by renin).
  c. True. Pulmonary capillaries produce angiotensin converting enzyme.
  d. **Correct.** The heart is not involved in the renin-angiotensin-aldosterone system.
  REF: Page 245

25.
  a. **Correct.** Increased blood pressure is a feature of the fight or flight response.
  b. False. Increased metabolic rate is a feature of the fight or flight response.
  c. False. Dilation of the pupils is a feature of the fight or flight response.
  d. False.
  REF: Page 243

26.
  a. False. Alpha cells of the pancreatic islets secrete glucagon.
  b. **Correct.** Beta cells of the pancreatic islets secrete insulin.
  c. False. Delta cells of the pancreatic islets secrete somatostatin.
  d. False. Sympathetic nerve endings in the adrenal medulla release mainly noradrenaline.
  REF: Page 246

27.
  a. False. Insulin is a polypeptide hormone consisting of about 50 amino acids.
  b. False. Insulin decreases glycogenolysis (breakdown of glycogen into glucose).
  c. **Correct.** Insulin increases uptake of glucose into cells.
  d. False. Insulin secretion is inhibited by cortisol.
  REF: Page 246

28.
   a. False.
   b. False.
   c. False. Type 2 diabetes mellitus usually affects adults, and only sometimes requires treatment with insulin injections.
   d. **Correct.** Type 2 diabetes mellitus will already have caused long-term complications in 25% of patients at the time of diagnosis.
   REF: Page 255, Table 9.5

29.
   a. **Correct.**
   b. False.
   c. False.
   d. False.
   REF: Page 247, Table 9.4

30.
   a. False.
   b. False.
   c. **Correct.** Histamine is released from mast cells during inflammatory and allergic responses.
   d. False.
   REF: Page 248

CHAPTER 10

The Respiratory System

Feedback

1.
  a. **Correct.** Along with the perpendicular plate of the ethmoid bone and the cartilage of the nose, the vomer forms part of the nasal septum.
  b. False.
  c. False.
  d. False.
  REF: Figure 10.2

2.
  a. False.
  b. **Correct.** The anterior nares are the visible openings into the nose, and the posterior nares are the openings from the back of each nasal cavity into the pharynx.
  c. False.
  d. False.
  REF: Figure 10.3

3.
  a. False. The conchae extend from the ethmoid bone.
  b. and c. False. The conchae do neither, but increase the internal surface area of the nasal cavities and generate turbulence in the inhaled air, allowing more efficient warming and humidification.
  d. **Correct.**
  REF: Page 263

4.
  a. False.
  b. False.
  c. **Correct.**
  d. False.
  REF: Figure 10.4

5.
  a. False.
  b. **Correct.** Also called the Eustachian tubes, the auditory tubes link the pharynx with the air-filled middle ear and allow the air pressure in the middle ear to equalise with atmospheric pressures, protecting the tympanic membrane.
  c. False.
  d. False.
  REF: Page 264, Figures 10.4 and 8.1

6.

    a. False. The epiglottis is the leaf-shaped cartilage that acts as the lid of the laryngeal box, lifting and lowering as required to prevent food and liquids from entering the trachea.

    b. **Correct.** The cricoid cartilage is a ring-shaped cartilage, lying immediately below the thyroid cartilage and attached to it by the cricothyroid ligament.

    c. False. The paired, pyramid-shaped arytenoid cartilages lie posteriorly and form part of the posterior wall of the larynx.

    d. False. The thyroid cartilage (Adam's apple) encircles the laryngeal opening, but is much broader at the front than at the back.

    REF: Figure 10.6

7.

    a. **Correct.**

    b. False. Influenza is caused by the influenza virus.

    c. False. Allergic rhinitis is a hypersensitivity reaction, not an infection.

    d. False. Diphtheria is a bacterial infection caused by *Corynebacterium diphtheriae*.

    REF: Page 284

8.

    a. False. Relaxation of the muscles controlling the vocal cords allows them to separate, opening the glottis (the space between the vocal cords).

    b. **Correct.** Relaxation of the muscles controlling the vocal cords allows them to separate, permitting air to flow through the larynx.

    c. False. Relaxation of the muscles controlling the vocal cords reduces their tension, and the sounds produced when they vibrate is lower pitched.

    d. False. Relaxation of the vocal cords allows them to separate (abduct).

    REF: Page 267

9.

    a. False.

    b. **Correct.**

    c. False.

    d. False.

    REF: Page 268

10.

    a. False.

    b. **Correct.**

    c. False.

    d. False.

    REF: Figure 10.11

11.

    a. **Correct.**

    b. False. The glottis must be closed to allow pressure to build.

    c. False. The abdominal muscles contract, increasing intraabdominal pressure, which in turn increases thoracic pressure and aids coughing.

    d. False. Immediately prior to the cough action, there is a deep inspiration to fill the lungs and increase pressure.

    REF: Page 270

12.

    a. False. The costal surfaces lie against the ribs.

    b. False. It is covered by the visceral pleura.

    c. **Correct.** The medial surfaces face one another across the mediastinum.

    d. False. The intercostal muscles lie between the ribs.

    REF: Page 271

13.
    a. **Correct.** There is only one pulmonary artery supplying each lung.
    b. False.
    c. False.
    d. False.
    REF: Figure 10.16

14.
    a. False.
    b. False.
    c. False.
    d. **Correct.**
    REF: Figure 10.15

15.
    a. False. The healthy lung contains little fibrous tissue.
    b. **Correct.** The elastic tissue allows the lung to expand and recoil during breathing.
    c. False. Only the larger airways contain cartilage, for support.
    d. False. There is no adipose tissue in the lung substance.
    REF: Page 274

16.
    a. False. The respiratory epithelium lines the upper respiratory tract.
    b. False. The visceral pleura covers the lung surface.
    c. **Correct.** The respiratory membrane comprises the alveolar wall and the capillary wall.
    d. False. The parietal pleura adheres to the inside of the ribcage.
    REF: Page 280, Figure 10.24A

17.
    a. False. The right lung has three lobes, the left only two.
    b. **Correct.** The right lung is displaced upwards in the chest because of the bulky liver below.
    c. False. The left lung is smaller than the right.
    d. False. This applies to both lungs.
    REF: Figure 10.13

18.
    a. False. Atopic (extrinsic) asthma is usually diagnosed in childhood.
    b. False. Atopic asthma is strongly associated with allergy, e.g., eczema and hay fever, both in the affected individual and in family members.
    c. **Correct.** There is a clear hereditable tendency in atopic asthma.
    d. False. Asthma is associated with bronchoconstriction.
    REF: Page 287

19.
    a. False.
    b. False.
    c. False.
    d. **Correct.**
    REF: Page 274

20.
    a. False. Pneumothorax is a cause of lung collapse, but refers specifically to air in the pleural space.
    b. **Correct.**
    c. False. Emphysema can cause lung collapse, but refers to destruction of alveolar walls, which produces large cavities in the lung tissue.
    d. False. Pleurisy is inflammation of the pleura.
    REF: Page 292

21.
    a. **Correct.**
    b. False.
    c. False.
    d. False.
    REF: Page 274
22.
    a. False.
    b. **Correct.**
    c. False.
    d. False.
    REF: Page 280
23.
    a. False.
    b. **Correct.**
    c. False.
    d. False.
    REF: Page 275
24.
    a. False. The diaphragm is the main respiratory muscle.
    b. False. The external intercostals are used during quiet breathing.
    c. False. The deltoid is not used in respiration.
    d. **Correct.** The internal intercostals help in forced expiration.
    REF: Page 276
25.
    a. False. The phrenic nerve stimulates contraction of the diaphragm.
    b. **Correct.**
    c. False. The diaphragm forms the roof of the abdominal cavity.
    d. False. When its fibres contract, the diaphragm sinks, lengthening the thoracic cavity.
    REF: Page 276, Figure 5.27
26.
    a. False. The intrapleural space is a potential space between the visceral and parietal pleura.
    b. False. There are between 7 and 10 mL of pleural fluid in the pleural space.
    c. **Correct.** This negative pressure holds the pleura together and keeps the lung expanded.
    d. False. This describes the mediastinum.
    REF: Page 272
27.
    a. False.
    b. False.
    c. False.
    d. **Correct.**
    REF: Figure 10.23
28.
    a. **Correct.**
    b. False.
    c. False.
    d. False.
    REF: Page 279, Table 10.1

29.
  a. False.
  b. False.
  c. **Correct.**
  d. False.
  REF: Figure 10.24
30.
  a. False. The partial pressure of oxygen (PO_2) of pulmonary venous blood is much higher than in the pulmonary artery, as it has been oxygenated in the pulmonary capillaries.
  b. False. The PO_2 of aortic blood is much higher than in the pulmonary artery, as it has been oxygenated in the pulmonary capillaries.
  c. **Correct.** Venous blood leaving the tissues is pumped to the lungs for oxygenation.
  d. False. The PO_2 of blood in the pulmonary artery and the PO_2 of blood in the vena cava are the same.
  REF: Page 280
31.
  a. False.
  b. **Correct.** The remainder is carried bound reversibly to haemoglobin.
  c. False.
  d. False.
  REF: Page 281
32.
  a. False. Regular firing of inspiratory neurones in the respiratory centre sets the basic rhythm of breathing.
  b. False. Expiratory neurones fire to help in forced expiration.
  c. False. There are stretch receptors in the lung tissue to prevent overinflation of the lungs, but the pneumotaxic area is in the brainstem.
  d. **Correct.**
  REF: Page 281
33.
  a. False. Falling blood pressure stimulates respiratory effort, to try to maintain oxygen supply to the tissues.
  b. False. Increased blood oxygen levels reduce respiratory effort.
  c. **Correct.** Decreased blood pH reflects rising blood carbon dioxide levels, and stimulates respiratory effort.
  d. False. Reduced blood H^+ reflects reduced blood acidity (rising pH), and reduces respiratory effort.
  REF: Page 281

CHAPTER 11

Introduction to Nutrition

Feedback

1.
   a. False.
   b. False.
   c. **Correct.** Non-starch polysaccharides are not nutrients because they are not essential for cellular metabolism and do not provide energy; however, they are an important dietary constituent.
   d. False.
   REF: Page 297

2.
   a. False.
   b. **Correct.** BMI between 18.5 and 24.9 is within the normal range.
   c. False.
   d. False.
   REF: Page 298, Box 11.1

3.
   a. False.
   b. False.
   c. **Correct.** BMI between 25.0 and 29.9 is overweight.
   d. False.
   REF: Page 298, Box 11.1

4.
   a. **Correct.** Fats release most energy per gram.
   b. False.
   c. False.
   d. False.
   REF: Page 299

5.
   a. False.
   b. False.
   c. **Correct.** Sweet potatoes are starchy carbohydrates.
   d. False.
   REF: Page 298

6.
   a. False.
   b. **Correct.**
   c. False.
   d. False.
   REF: Page 301

7.
    a. **Correct.** Both saturated and unsaturated fats are also known as triglycerides.
    b. False. Saturated fats come from animal sources.
    c. False. Saturated fats are usually solid at room temperature.
    d. False. Fats consist of carbon, hydrogen and oxygen, but unlike carbohydrates, the hydrogen and oxygen are not the same proportions as water.
    REF: Page 301

8.
    a. False.
    b. False.
    c. False.
    d. **Correct.**
    REF: Page 299

9.
    a. **Correct.**
    b. False. Vitamins B and C are water soluble.
    c. False.
    d. False.
    REF: Page 302

10.
    a. **Correct.**
    b. False.
    c. False.
    d. False. Sodium, potassium and calcium are all required for contraction of muscle.
    REF: Pages 304 and 305

11.
    a. False.
    b. False.
    c. **Correct.**
    d. False.
    REF: Page 300

12.
    a. **Correct.**
    b. False. Low-density lipoproteins are harmful to health when blood levels are excessive.
    c. False.
    d. False.
    REF: Page 302

13.
    a. False.
    b. False.
    c. False.
    d. **Correct.** More iron is needed to compensate for blood loss during menstruation.
    REF: Page 305

14.
    a. False.
    b. **Correct.** Iodine is sometimes added to table salt in small amounts to prevent goitre.
    c. False.
    d. False.
    REF: Page 305

15.
  a. False.
  b. False.
  c. False.
  d. **Correct.** Vitamin B_{12} is needed for DNA synthesis. Deficiency is usually associated with insufficient intrinsic factor (secreted by the stomach) that is essential for its absorption.
  REF: Page 304
16.
  a. False. Deficiency becomes apparent after 4–6 months.
  b. False. Niacin is vitamin B_3.
  c. False. Vitamin C is water soluble.
  d. **Correct.** Vitamin C is easily destroyed, e.g., by cooking, salting, chopping and drying.
  REF: Page 304
17.
  a. False.
  b. False.
  c. False.
  d. **Correct.**
  REF: Page 302
18.
  a. False.
  b. **Correct.**
  c. False.
  d. False.
  REF: Page 307
19.
  a. **Correct.**
  b. False.
  c. False.
  d. False. Kwashiorkor is associated with liver damage, causing reduced plasma proteins leading to oedema, and it is often precipitated by infections such as measles or gastroenteritis.
  REF: Page 307, Figure 11.2
20.
  a. False.
  b. False.
  c. **Correct.**
  d. False.
  REF: Page 308

CHAPTER 12

The Digestive System

Feedback

1.

   a. **Correct.** The physiological term for eating and drinking is ingestion.

   b. False. Propulsion is mixing and movement of the contents along the alimentary tract.

   c. False. Absorption is the process by which digested food substances pass through the walls of some organs into the circulation.

   d. False. Digestion consists of mechanical breakdown and chemical digestion of food.

   REF: Page 312

2.

   a. True. The mucosa is the innermost layer.

   b. True. The submucosa lies outside the mucosa.

   c. True. The serosa forms the outermost layer of the alimentary tract wall.

   d. **Correct.** All of the layers above are present in the walls of the alimentary tract.

   REF: Page 314

3.

   a. False.

   b. False.

   c. **Correct.** The duodenum is not an accessory organ of digestion, it is part of the digestive tract.

   d. False.

   REF: Page 314

4.

   a. False. The visceral peritoneum covers abdominal and pelvic organs.

   b. **Correct.** The parietal peritoneum lines the abdominal wall.

   c. False. The mesentery is a double fold of visceral peritoneum that attaches the stomach and intestines to the posterior abdominal wall.

   d. False. The greater omentum is formed from the fold of peritoneum that encloses the stomach and hangs down in front of it.

   REF: Page 314, Figure 12.3

5.

   a. False.

   b. False.

   c. **Correct.** The kidneys are retroperitoneal (lie behind the peritoneum).

   d. False.

   REF: Pages 314 and 315

6.
    a. False. The circular muscle fibres lie inside the longitudinal fibres.
    b. False. The plexus lies between the two muscle layers.
    c. False. Peristalsis requires contraction and relaxation of both the circular and longitudinal muscle fibres
    d. **Correct.** Sphincters are rings of thickened circular muscle.
    REF: Page 315

7.
    a. False.
    b. False.
    c. **Correct.** The myenteric plexus contains sympathetic and parasympathetic nerves that supply the muscle layer and is located between the circular and longitudinal fibres.
    d. False.
    REF: Page 315, Figure 12.2

8.
    a. True. Parasympathetic stimulation increases muscular activity, especially peristalsis, through stimulation of the myenteric plexus.
    b. True. Glandular secretion is increased through stimulation of the submucosal plexus.
    c. **Correct.** Parasympathetic stimulation of the alimentary tract increases both muscular activity and glandular secretion.
    d. False.
    REF: Page 317

9.
    a. **Correct.**
    b. False.
    c. False.
    d. False.
    REF: Page 316, Figure 12.5

10.
    a. False.
    b. False.
    c. False.
    d. **Correct.** The oesophagus is not a boundary of the oral cavity. The oral cavity is bounded by the lips anteriorly, the palate superiorly, the tongue inferiorly and is continuous with the oropharynx posteriorly.
    REF: Page 318

11.
    a. **Correct.** The hypoglossal nerve supplies the voluntary muscles of tongue.
    b. False. The lingual branch of mandibular nerve is the nerve of somatic sensation, i.e., pain, temperature and touch.
    c. False.
    d. False. The facial and glossopharyngeal nerves are involved in taste.
    REF: Page 319

12.
    a. True.
    b. True.
    c. True.
    d. **Correct.** The sensory receptors (nerve endings) of taste are present in the papillae and widely distributed in the epithelium of the tongue, soft palate, pharynx and epiglottis.
    REF: Page 319

13.
  a. False. The deciduous teeth begin to erupt at the age of 6 months.
  b. **Correct.** All deciduous teeth should be present by the age of 24 months.
  c. False. The permanent teeth begin to replace the deciduous teeth at 6 years.
  d. False. The permanent dentition is usually complete by 21 years.
  REF: Page 319, Table 12.1
14.
  a. False. The pulp cavity is in the centre of the tooth and contains the blood vessels, lymph vessels and nerves.
  b. False. Dentine is the hard ivory-like substance surrounding the pulp cavity.
  c. False. The dentine is covered by a thin layer enamel.
  d. **Correct.** The root of a tooth is covered by a substance resembling bone, called cementum, which secures it in its socket.
  REF: Page 319, Figure 12.12
15.
  a. **Correct.** The parotid ducts open into the mouth beside the second upper molar tooth.
  b. False. The submandibular ducts open onto the floor of the mouth, one on each side of the frenulum of the tongue.
  c. False. The sublingual ducts open into the floor of the mouth.
  d. False. The adrenal glands are not salivary glands; they lie above each kidney.
  REF: Pages 320 and 321
16.
  a. False. The tongue is supplied by the lingual branch of the external carotid artery.
  b. False. The teeth are supplied by branches of the maxillary arteries.
  c. **Correct.** The pharynx is supplied by several branches of the facial arteries.
  d. False. The oesophagus is supplied by branches from the thoracic aorta, inferior phrenic arteries and left gastric branch of coeliac artery.
  REF: Pages 318, 320 and 322
17.
  a. False.
  b. **Correct.** The oesophagus passes between muscle fibres of the diaphragm behind the central tendon at the level of the 10th thoracic vertebra.
  c. False.
  d. False.
  REF: Page 322, Figure 12.10
18.
  a. **Correct.**
  b. False.
  c. False.
  d. False.
  REF: Page 348, Table 12.4
19.
  a. True.
  b. True.
  c. True.
  d. **Correct.** All of the above are responsible for minimising gastric reflux.
  REF: Page 322

20.

    a. False.

    b. **Correct.** The stomach has three layers (longitudinal, circular and oblique) of muscle fibres.

    c. False.

    d. False. The oesophagus and small and large intestines all have two layers of muscle fibres.

    REF: Page 325, Figure 12.19

21.

    a. False. Mucous neck cells secrete mucus.

    b. False. Parietal cells secrete hydrochloric acid and intrinsic factor.

    c. **Correct.** Chief cells secrete pepsinogen.

    d. False.

    REF: Page 326

22.

    a. **Correct.**

    b. False.

    c. False.

    d. False.

    REF: Pages 358 and 359, Figure 12.52

23.

    a. False. The cephalic phase involves secretion of gastric juice before food reaches the stomach.

    b. False. Gastrin is secreted in the gastric phase.

    c. **Correct.** Secretin and cholecystokinin are secreted in the intestinal phase.

    d. False.

    REF: Page 328, Figure 12.22

24.

    a. False. A carbohydrate-rich meal leaves the stomach in 2–3 h.

    b. False. A protein-rich meal remains longer than carbohydrate meal.

    c. **Correct.** A fatty meal remains in the stomach for longest.

    d. False.

    REF: Page 328

25.

    a. False. Vomiting is a reflex (involuntary) process.

    b. **Correct.**

    c. False. Vomiting can lead to serious alkalosis if severe (caused by loss of hydrochloric acid in vomit).

    d. False. Vomiting is coordinated by the medulla.

    REF: Page 348, Table 12.4

26.

    a. False. The large intestine is 1.5 m in length.

    b. False. The duodenum is 25 cm in length.

    c. False. The jejunum is 2 m in length.

    d. **Correct.** The ileum is the longest, at about 3 m.

    REF: Page 328

27.

    a. **Correct.**

    b. False. In ulcerative colitis the rectum is always involved with variable spread along the colon.

    c. False.

    d. False. Ulcerative colitis affects the mucosa rather than the whole thickness of the intestinal wall and ulcers and fistulae are also typical of Crohn's disease, not ulcerative colitis.

    REF: Page 357 and Table 12.5

28.
 a. False. The stomach empties through the pyloric sphincter.
 b. **Correct.** The duodenal papilla is guarded by a ring of smooth muscle, the hepatopancreatic sphincter (of Oddi).
 c. False. There are no sphincters in the jejunum.
 d. False. The ileum ends at ileocecal valve.
 REF: Page 328

29.
 a. False.
 b. False.
 c. **Correct.** The distal end of ileum has collections of larger lymph nodes called aggregated lymphoid follicles (Peyer's patches).
 d. False.
 REF: Page 330, Figure 12.25

30.
 a. False.
 b. **Correct.** The epithelium of the entire small intestine is replaced every 3–5 days.
 c. False.
 d. False.
 REF: Page 330

31.
 a. False.
 b. False.
 c. False.
 d. **Correct.** Barrett's oesophagus is regarded as a premalignant condition.
 REF: Page 351

32.
 a. **Correct.** Trypsinogen is an inactive enzyme precursor present in pancreatic juice.
 b. False. Cholecystokinin is a hormone secreted by the small intestine.
 c. False.
 d. False. Intrinsic factor and pepsinogen are constituents of gastric juice.
 REF: Page 331

33.
 a. False. Hepatitis B is spread by contaminated blood, body fluids and blood products.
 b. **Correct.**
 c. False.
 d. False. Hepatitis B has an incubation period of 50–180 days and is usually a severe illness.
 REF: Page 362

34.
 a. False.
 b. False.
 c. **Correct.** Vitamin D is fat soluble and absorbed into lacteals with lipids.
 d. False. Vitamins B, C and folic acid are water soluble and are therefore absorbed into the capillaries in the villi.
 REF: Page 332

35.

   a. False. Intrinsic factor required for vitamin B_{12} absorption is secreted in the stomach.

   b. False.

   c. **Correct.** Vitamin B_{12} combines with intrinsic factor in the stomach and is actively absorbed in the terminal ileum.

   d. False.

   REF: Page 332

36.

   a. False.

   b. **Correct.** The sigmoid colon located in the pelvic cavity has an S-shaped curve.

   c. False.

   d. False.

   REF: Page 333

37.

   a. False.

   b. False.

   c. False.

   d. **Correct.** The anal canal is a short passage about 3.8 cm long in adults.

   REF: Page 333

38.

   a. **Correct.** The superior mesenteric artery supplies the caecum, ascending colon and most of the transverse colon.

   b. False. The inferior mesenteric artery supplies the remainder of the colon.

   c. False.

   d. False. The middle and inferior rectal arteries supply the distal section of the rectum and anus.

   REF: Page 335

39.

   a. False.

   b. **Correct.** The liver is the largest gland in the body, weighing between 1 and 2.3 kg.

   c. False.

   d. False.

   REF: Page 336

40.

   a. **Correct.**

   b. False.

   c. False.

   d. False.

   REF: Page 337

41.

   a. True.

   b. True.

   c. True.

   d. **Correct.** The liver is related to the diaphragm anteriorly, posteriorly and laterally.

   REF: Page 337

42.
  a. True.
  b. True.
  c. **Correct.** Both cholic and chenodeoxycholic acids are bile acids synthesised by hepatocytes from cholesterol.
  d. False.
  REF: Page 339

43.
  a. False.
  b. **Correct.**
  c. False.
  d. False.
  REF: Page 339

44.
  a. **Correct.** Viral hepatitis is a cause of intrahepatic jaundice
  b. False. Impacted gallstones are a cause of posthepatic jaundice.
  c. False. Excessive haemolysis is a cause of prehepatic jaundice.
  d. False. A tumour of the head of the pancreas causes posthepatic jaundice.
  REF: Page 365

45.
  a. False. The right and left hepatic ducts merge just after leaving the portal fissure.
  b. False. The hepatic duct is joined by the cystic duct from the gallbladder.
  c. False. The right and left hepatic ducts merge forming the common hepatic duct.
  d. **Correct.**
  REF: Page 340, Figure 12.38

46.
  a. False.
  b. False.
  c. **Correct.**
  d. False.
  REF: Page 365, Figure 12.54

47.
  a. True.
  b. True.
  c. True.
  d. **Correct.** All of the above are functions of gallbladder.
  REF: Page 341

48.
  a. False.
  b. False.
  c. False. Metabolic rate is higher in men than women and decreases with age and during starvation.
  d. **Correct.**
  REF: Page 342, Table 12.3

49.
  a. False.
  b. False.
  c. **Correct.**
  d. False. Glycolysis, the citric acid cycle and oxidative phosphorylation are the three central metabolic pathways.
  REF: Pages 343–346

50.
   a. False.
   b. **Correct.** Glycolysis does not require oxygen and is therefore an anaerobic pathway.
   c. False.
   d. False.
   REF: Page 344

CHAPTER 13

The Urinary System

Feedback

1.

    a. False. The right lobe of the liver lies anteriorly to the right kidney.

    b. False. The duodenum lies anteriorly to the right kidney.

    c. False. The hepatic flexure of the colon lies anteriorly to the right kidney.

    d. **Correct.** The pancreas lies anteriorly to the left kidney.

    REF: Page 370

2.

    a. False. The capsule is the outer fibrous covering that surrounds the kidney.

    b. False. The cortex is the reddish-brown layer of tissue immediately below the capsule.

    c. False. The medulla is the innermost layer consisting of renal pyramids.

    d. **Correct.** The hilum is the concave medial border of the kidney where the renal blood and lymph vessels, ureter and nerves enter.

    REF: Page 371

3.

    a. False.

    b. False.

    c. **Correct.** The renal pelvis is the funnel-shaped structure that collects urine formed by the kidney.

    d. False.

    REF: Page 371

4.

    a. **Correct.** The functional unit of the kidney is the nephron.

    b. False.

    c. False.

    d. False.

    REF: Page 371

5.

    a. False.

    b. **Correct.** The kidneys receive about 20% of the cardiac output.

    c. False.

    d. False.

    REF: Page 371

6.
   a. **Correct.** The afferent arteriole enters each glomerular capsule and then subdivides into a cluster of tiny arterial capillaries, forming the glomerulus.
   b. False. The efferent arteriole is the blood vessel leading away from the glomerulus.
   c. False. The afferent arteriole is larger in diameter than the efferent arteriole, which increases the hydrostatic pressure inside the glomerulus, driving filtration across the glomerular capillary walls.
   d. False. The efferent arteriole divides forming the peritubular capillary network that allows exchange of substances between the tubules and the bloodstream.
   REF: Page 371

7.
   a. True. Filtration occurs in the glomerulus.
   b. True.
   c. True. Selective reabsorption and secretion occur in the convoluted tubules.
   d. **Correct.** All of the above are involved in formation of urine.
   REF: Pages 373 and 374

8.
   a. True.
   b. True.
   c. True. Water, glucose and creatinine are normal constituents of glomerular filtrate.
   d. **Correct.** Plasma proteins are not a normal constituent of glomerular filtrate.
   REF: Page 374, Box 13.1

9.
   a. False.
   b. **Correct.** In healthy adults the GFR is about 125 mL/min, i.e., 180 L of filtrate is formed each day by the two kidneys.
   c. False.
   d. False.
   REF: Page 374

10.
   a. **Correct.** Parathyroid hormone does not influence reabsorption of sodium or water; it regulates reabsorption of calcium and phosphate.
   b. True. Antidiuretic hormone increases water reabsorption.
   c. True. Aldosterone increases reabsorption of sodium and water, and excretion of potassium.
   d. True. Atrial natriuretic peptide decreases reabsorption of sodium and water.
   REF: Page 375

11.
   a. False. The specific gravity of urine is between 1020 and 1030.
   b. **Correct.** The pH of urine is around 6.
   c. False. Adults normally pass 1000–1500 mL urine per day.
   d. False. Urine is 96% water.
   REF: Page 375

12.
   a. False.
   b. **Correct.** In order to maintain normal blood pH (acid–base balance), the proximal convoluted tubules secrete hydrogen ions into the filtrate.
   c. False.
   d. False.
   REF: Page 377

13.
    a. **Correct.** Sodium is the most common cation in extracellular fluid.
    b. False.
    c. False.
    d. False.
    REF: Page 376

14.
    a. True. Electrolytes excreted in sweat are increased in pyrexia (fever).
    b. True. High environmental temperature increases electrolyte loss in sweat.
    c. True. Sustained physical exercise increases electrolyte loss in sweat.
    d. **Correct.** All of the above are associated with an increased loss of electrolytes, including sodium, in sweat.
    REF: Page 376

15.
    a. False. The lungs produce angiotensin converting enzyme (ACE), which converts angiotensin 1 into angiotensin 2.
    b. **Correct.** The plasma protein angiotensinogen is produced by the liver.
    c. False. The proximal convoluted tubules of the nephrons produce ACE, which converts angiotensin 1 into angiotensin 2.
    d. False. The adrenal cortex secretes the hormone aldosterone, which regulates the amount of sodium excreted in the urine.
    REF: Page 377

16.
    a. False.
    b. **Correct.** Deficiency of erythropoietin, the hormone that stimulates erythropoiesis, leads to anaemia.
    c. False.
    d. False.
    REF: Page 386

17.
    a. False.
    b. False.
    c. **Correct.** The total capacity of the bladder is about 600 mL.
    d. False.
    REF: Page 379

18.
    a. False.
    b. **Correct.** When the bladder contains 300–400 mL of urine, awareness of the need to pass urine is normally felt.
    c. False.
    d. False.
    REF: Page 381

19.
    a. False. Passing large volumes of urine is known as polyuria.
    b. False. Passing urine during the night is known as nocturia.
    c. False. Urine output less than 400 mL/day is oliguria.
    d. **Correct.** Dysuria is pain on passing urine
    REF: Page 383, Table 13.1

20.

   a. **Correct.** Cystitis is associated with frequency of micturition.
   b. False. Cystitis is more common in females than males because of the shorter urethra.
   c. False. Cystitis is not always associated with infection; it can also be caused by trauma, e.g., radiotherapy or insertion of instruments into the bladder.
   d. False. Cystitis is inflammation of the bladder.
   REF: Page 389

CHAPTER 14

The Skin

Feedback

1.
    a. False.
    b. False.
    c. **Correct.**
    d. False.
    REF: Page 393

2.
    a. **Correct.**
    b. False. The epidermis lies above the dermis.
    c. False. The epidermis does not contain nerve endings or blood vessels.
    d. False. The epidermis is replaced in 1 month.
    REF: Page 393

3.
    a. False.
    b. False.
    c. False.
    d. **Correct.** Keratin replaces the cytoplasm in the flattened cells on the skin surface.
    REF: Page 394

4.
    a. **Correct.**
    b. False. Areolar and adipose tissue are found in the subcutaneous layer of the skin.
    c. False. The ducts of sweat glands open onto the dermis.
    d. False. The epidermis varies in thickness according to the amount of wear and tear an area is subject to.
    REF: Page 395

5.
    a. False.
    b. False.
    c. **Correct.**
    d. False.
    REF: Page 395, Table 14.1

6.
    a. False.
    b. **Correct.**
    c. False.
    d. False.
    REF: Page 396

7.
    a. False. Sebum protects the skin from maceration.
    b. False. The arrector pili muscles enable skin hairs to stand erect.
    c. False. Dendritic cells play no role in temperature regulation.
    d. **Correct.**
    REF: Page 397

8.
    a. False.
    b. False.
    c. False.
    d. **Correct.** Melanin is secreted by melanocytes in the deep germinative layer of the epidermis; its synthesis is stimulated by exposure to sunlight.
    REF: Pages 395 and 397

9.
    a. False. Heat loss occurs by conduction when clothes in direct contact with the skin take up heat
    b. **Correct.**
    c. False. Small amounts of heat are also lost in expired air, urine and faeces.
    d. False. Heat loss increases when there is vasodilation.
    REF: Pages 397 and 398

10.
    a. False.
    b. False.
    c. False.
    d. **Correct.** Wearing several layers of clothes will reduce heat loss but does not affect generation of heat.
    REF: Page 397

11.
    a. **Correct.**
    b. False. Body temperature is controlled by the temperature regulating centre in the hypothalamus.
    c. False. Body temperature is under negative feedback control.
    d. False. Body temperature rises in women just after ovulation.
    REF: Pages 397 and 398

12.
    a. False. Vasodilation of the arterioles in the skin allows more blood flow there.
    b. **Correct.** The skin is pink in colour and warm to touch when body temperature is elevated.
    c. False. The temperature regulation centre responds to changes in temperature of the circulating blood.
    d. False. Chemicals known as pyrogens reset the thermostat in the hypothalamus to a higher level.
    REF: Page 398

13.
    a. False.
    b. False.
    c. **Correct.**
    d. False.
    REF: Page 398

14.
  a. **Correct.** Surgical incisions normally heal by first intention because there is minimal tissue loss and the edges are in close apposition.
  b. False. Any bacteria present are removed by phagocytes.
  c. False. The first stage is the inflammatory phase.
  d. False. Fibroblasts secrete new collagen fibres
  REF: Page 399
15.
  a. False.
  b. False.
  c. False.
  d. **Correct.**
  REF: Page 401, Figure 14.10
16.
  a. False.
  b. **Correct.** As the germinative layer becomes less active, the epidermis thins.
  c. False.
  d. False.
  REF: Page 402
17.
  a. False. Herpes zoster is responsible for shingles and chicken pox.
  b. **Correct.**
  c. False. *Staphylococcus aureus* causes impetigo.
  d. False. *Streptococcus pyogenes* is a cause of cellulitis.
  REF: Page 403
18.
  a. False.
  b. False.
  c. **Correct.**
  d. False. Psoriasis is sometimes associated with rheumatoid arthritis.
  REF: Page 403
19.
  a. False. Burns are first degree when only the **epidermis** is affected.
  b. **Correct.** Burns are relatively painless when they are full thickness because the sensory nerve endings in the dermis will have been destroyed.
  c. False. Burns can only heal by secondary intention when they are full thickness and will usually require skin grafting.
  d. False. Burns may be complicated by hypovolaemic shock when 15% of the body surface is affected.
  REF: Pages 404 and 405
20.
  a. **Correct.** Basal cell carcinoma is associated with long-term exposure to sunlight. Although it is malignant, it is different from a malignant melanoma and seldom metastasises.
  b. False.
  c. False.
  d. False.
  REF: Page 405

CHAPTER 15

Introduction to Immunity

Feedback

1.
   a. False. Innate immunity refers to non-specific defences with which the individual is born, such as gastric acid and inflammation.
   b. **Correct.** Specific defence learns and adapts according to the antigens to which it is exposed.
   c. False. This term is not used in immune biology.
   d. False. Immunological surveillance belongs to the innate immune system and is non-specific.
   REF: Page 407

2.
   a. False. Cilia sweep mucus away from the lungs in the respiratory tract, but villi are not motile: their function is in absorption.
   b. False. Intact skin is a very effective barrier, but its surface is not sterile: it is heavily colonised by (usually) non-pathogenic commensal bacteria.
   c. **Correct.**
   d. False. Lysozyme is an antibacterial enzyme found in body fluids, e.g. tears and saliva.
   REF: Page 408

3.
   a. **Correct.** Complement performs several protective functions, including attracting phagocytes.
   b. False. An immune complex is produced by combination of antibody and antigen molecules.
   c. False. Immunoglobulins are also known as antibodies.
   d. False. Complement is part of the host defences, not a bacterial protein.
   REF: Page 409

4.
   a. False.
   b. False.
   c. **Correct.**
   d. False.
   REF: Page 409

5.
   a. False.
   b. False.
   c. False.
   d. **Correct.** Interleukin 1, released by white blood cells in response to infection, resets the temperature regulatory centre in the hypothalamus and triggers fever.
   REF: Page 411

6.
  a. False.
  b. False.
  c. **Correct.**
  d. False.
  REF: Page 411

7.
  a. False. Phagocytes are part of the innate, non-specific response.
  b. **Correct.** Tolerance means the adaptive immune system recognises and tolerates 'self' tissues.
  c. False. Adaptive immunity is specific immunity.
  d. False. Immunological surveillance is part of the innate, non-specific defence system.
  REF: Page 407

8.
  a. False. This applies to both T- and B-cells.
  b. False. This applies to both T- and B-cells.
  c. **Correct.**
  d. False. This applies to both T- and B-cells.
  REF: Page 412

9.
  a. False. Antigen presenting cells (APCs) are non-specific, i.e. they ingest and present any antigenic material.
  b. False. Plasma cells, derived from B-cells, produce antibodies.
  c. False. APCs trigger clonal expansion in T-cells when they present antigen to them, but do not themselves undergo clonal expansion.
  d. **Correct.**
  REF: Page 412

10.
  a. **Correct.** Regulatory T-cells (T-regs) suppress the immune system once an infection has been controlled.
  b. False. T-regs suppress other immune cells.
  c. False. Memory T-cells are the longest-lived subtype of T-cells.
  d. False. Plasma cells, derived from B-cells, make antibodies.
  REF: Page 413, Figure 15.3

11.
  a. False. Cytotoxic T-cells are only produced during active infection.
  b. **Correct.** Immunity to an infection is due to populations of fast-reacting memory B- and memory T-cells, generated during the original infection.
  c. False. Regulatory T-cells suppress the immune system after the infection has been dealt with and disappear after that.
  d. False. Helper T-cells are produced as part of the ongoing immune response but disappear after the infection has been resolved.
  REF: Page 413

12.
  a. False. Antibodies bind to bacteria and bacterial toxins.
  b. **Correct.** A B-cell uses its own antibody to detect the presence of specific antigen.
  c. False. Antibodies travel in the blood and readily enter the tissues and body fluids.
  d. False. Antibodies are globulins (immunoglobulins).
  REF: Page 414

13.

    a. False. IgG is present in large amounts in the secondary immune response.

    b. False. IgE is the immunoglobulin associated with allergy.

    c. **Correct.**

    d. False. IgA is found in most body secretions, including breast milk.

    REF: Page 414, Table 15.2

14.

    a. **Correct.**

    b. False. The primary immune response is characterised by high levels of IgM.

    c. False. Memory cells only appear following a primary immune response.

    d. False. The primary immune response is the response to (usually) the first exposure to an infection, whatever the causative organism.

    REF: Page 415, Figure 15.6

15.

    a. False.

    b. False.

    c. False.

    d. **Correct.**

    REF: Page 415, Figure 15.7

16.

    a. False. Macrophages, part of the innate defence system, arrive relatively quickly on the scene (peaking about a week post-infection), but both neutrophils and natural killer cells peak earlier than this.

    b. False. Cytotoxic T-cells, part of the adaptive immune system, peak over a week post-infection.

    c. **Correct.** Natural killer cells, part of the innate defence system, peak 2 or 3 days post-infection.

    d. False. Plasma cells, producing antibodies, can take up to 2 weeks to peak.

    REF: Page 416

17.

    a. False. The incidence of autoimmune disease does rise with age but is associated with reduced tolerance and the production of autoantibodies.

    b. **Correct.**

    c. False. Age-related immune decline can contribute to increased risk of infections, but this is not specifically related to natural killer cell decline.

    d. False. Older people often do suffer from fewer minor viral infections, e.g. colds, because they are likely to have been exposed to a wide range of viral strains in their lifetime.

    REF: Page 416

18.

    a. False. Type I hypersensitivity is usually called allergy and relates to excessive release of histamine in response to antigen exposure.

    b. **Correct.** Type II hypersensitivity is associated with the production of autoantibodies, causing autoimmune disease, e.g. rheumatoid arthritis.

    c. False. Type III hypersensitivity is associated with the abnormal generation and deposition of immune complexes, e.g. penicillin allergy.

    d. False. Type IV hypersensitivity is due to abnormal activation of T-cells, which destroy body tissues, e.g. graft rejection.

    REF: Page 417

19.

    a. False. It usually takes years for the virus to destroy enough immune cells to lead to significant immunocompromise.

    b. False. The virus can be isolated from most body fluids, including blood, semen, breast milk, cerebrospinal fluid and urine.

    c. **Correct.** HIV has only single-stranded RNA, and to infect host cells, this has to be converted into double-stranded DNA by the viral enzyme reverse transcriptase.

    d. False. The receptor subtype is CD_4, not CD_2.

REF: Page 419

20.

    a. **Correct.**

    b. False.

    c. False.

    d. False.

REF: Page 417, Table 15.3

The Musculoskeletal System

Feedback

1.
    a. False.
    b. **Correct.**
    c. False.
    d. False.
    REF: Page 422

2.
    a. False.
    b. False.
    c. False.
    d. **Correct.**
    REF: Page 422, Figure 16.1

3.
    a. **Correct.**
    b. False. The central medullary cavity is filled with yellow bone marrow.
    c. False. Periosteum is the outer, fibrous covering of the bone.
    d. False. Bone ends that form joints are covered with hyaline cartilage.
    REF: Page 422

4.
    a. False. Bone is about 2/3 calcium salts, but this is not osteoid.
    b. **Correct.** Osteoid is the organic component of bone and is mainly collagen.
    c. False. Bone cells comprise less than 2% of bone mass.
    d. False. Bone contains no elastic tissue.
    REF: Page 423

5.
    a. False.
    b. False.
    c. **Correct.**
    d. False.
    REF: Page 423

6.
    a. False.
    b. False.
    c. False.
    d. **Correct.** As mature bone cells, osteocytes live in these small cavities, surrounded by the bone that they have deposited around themselves.
    REF: Page 423

7.
  a. **Correct.** The central canal carries blood vessels to supply the cells of compact bone. In spongy bone tissue, cells are close enough to the surface of the bone for diffusion through canaliculi to supply their needs.
  b. False. Bone tissue is arranged in lamellae in both compact and spongy bone.
  c. False. Both compact and spongy bone contain canaliculi, the tiny channels linking adjacent lacunae.
  d. False. Both compact and spongy bone contain osteocytes living in lacunae.
  REF: Page 424

8.
  a. and b. False. Growth hormone and thyroxine stimulate bone growth during infancy and childhood.
  c. **Correct.** At puberty, oestrogen in the female and testosterone in males accelerates the deposition of bone in the epiphyseal plates, converting them completely to bone and making further lengthening of the bone impossible.
  d. False. Calcitonin increases the uptake of calcium into bone tissue.
  REF: Page 426

9.
  a. False.
  b. **Correct.**
  c. False.
  d. False.
  REF: Page 426

10.
  a. False.
  b. False.
  c. **Correct.**
  d. False.
  REF: Page 467

11.
  a. False.
  b. False.
  c. False.
  d. **Correct.**
  REF: Page 427, Table 16.1

12.
  a. False.
  b. False.
  c. **Correct.**
  d. False.
  REF: Page 428

13.
  a. False.
  b. False.
  c. False.
  d. **Correct.**
  REF: Page 426

14.
 a. **Correct.**
 b. False.
 c. False.
 d. False.
 REF: Page 429, Figure 16.10

15.
 a. False. The sphenoid bone forms part of the base of the skull, not the face.
 b. False. The cerebellum sits in the posterior cranial fossa of the occipital bone.
 c. **Correct.**
 d. False. The conchae are part of the nasal septum, and the sphenoid bone forms part of the base of the skull.
 REF: Page 431, Figure 16.15

16.
 a. **Correct.**
 b. False. The child may be 18 months old before the largest fontanelle is fully ossified.
 c. False. The fontanelles are easily palpable and obvious to visual inspection.
 d. False. The fontanelles' function is to allow some moulding of the skull bones during childbirth, to help the passage of the baby down the birth canal.
 REF: Pages 433 and 434

17.
 a. False. The atlas sits on top of the axis, and the bones are held together by the dens (odontoid process) of the axis projecting upwards into a ring formed by the transverse ligament of the atlas.
 b. **Correct.**
 c. False. The atlas sits on top of the axis, and has facets for the condyles of the occipital bone of the skull. This joint allows nodding of the head.
 d. False. The atlas does sit on top of the axis, but the joint between them allows the head to be turned from side to side.
 REF: Page 435, Figure 16.23

18.
 a. False.
 b. **Correct.** 24 separate vertebrae, plus the sacrum and the coccyx (each composed of fused vertebrae)
 c. False.
 d. False.
 REF: Page 434

19.
 a. False.
 b. False.
 c. False.
 d. **Correct.**
 REF: Page 434, Figure 16.20

20.
 a. False.
 b. False.
 c. **Correct.**
 d. False.
 REF: Page 440, Figure 16.34

21.
   a. **Correct.**
   b. False.
   c. False.
   d. False.
   REF: Page 441, Figure 16.36
22.
   a. False.
   b. False.
   c. **Correct.**
   d. False.
   REF: Page 442, Figure 16.37
23.
   a. False.
   b. **Correct.**
   c. False.
   d. False.
   REF: Page 444, Figure 16.42
24.
   a. False.
   b. False.
   c. False.
   d. **Correct.**
   REF: Page 446, Figure 16.45
25.
   a. False. Synovial joints are the most moveable joints, but limited movement is possible at some fibrous and cartilaginous joints as well.
   b. False. Sutures are fibrous joints.
   c. **Correct.**
   d. False. The joint capsule is lined with synovial membrane.
   REF: Page 446
26.
   a. False.
   b. **Correct.**
   c. False.
   d. False.
   REF: Page 447, Table 16.2 and Page 448, Figure 16.47
27.
   a. **Correct.**
   b. False.
   c. False.
   d. False.
   REF: Page 447
28.
   a. False.
   b. False.
   c. False.
   d. **Correct.**
   REF: Pages 448 and 450, Figure 16.49

29.
  a. False. There is a hereditable component, sometimes very strong.
  b. **Correct.**
  c. False. The disease usually appears first in the hands and feet.
  d. False. Pannus is inflammatory tissue laid down within the joint, which contributes to permanent deformity, pain and loss of function.
  REF: Page 470

30.
  a. False.
  b. **Correct.**
  c. False.
  d. False.
  REF: Page 446, Figure 16.46

31.
  a. False.
  b. False.
  c. False.
  d. **Correct.**
  REF: Page 449, Figure 16.48

32.
  a. False.
  b. False.
  c. **Correct.** The proximal radioulnar joint is a pivot joint formed as the annular ligament holds the head of the radius close to the ulna; the distal radioulnar joint is a pivot joint between the distal ends of the bones; the interosseous membrane is a fibrous joint, formed by a fibrous membrane holding the shafts of the bones together.
  d. False.
  REF: Page 449

33.
  a. False.
  b. False.
  c. False.
  d. **Correct.**
  REF: Page 451, Figure 16.51

34.
  a. False.
  b. False.
  c. **Correct.**
  d. False.
  REF: Page 452, Figure 16.52

35.
  a. False.
  b. **Correct.** The acetabulum is formed by the union of the three bones of the hip, and is the cavity in which the head of femur is held firmly by the ligamentum teres.
  c. False.
  d. False.
  REF: Pages 452 and 453, Figure 16.53

36.
a. **Correct.**
b. False.
c. False.
d. False.
REF: Page 453, Figure 16.54

37.
a. False.
b. False.
c. **Correct.**
d. False.
REF: Page 454

38.
a. False. Skeletal muscle cells are cylindrical.
b. False. Skeletal muscle cells are not supplied by autonomic nerves, but by somatic (voluntary) nerves.
c. **Correct.**
d. False. Skeletal muscle cells have multiple, peripheral nuclei.
REF: Page 455

39.
a. **Correct.** These three layers of connective tissue run from one end of the muscle to another, preventing overstretching, and form the tendon at each end of the muscle.
b. False. Ligaments, not tendons, fasten one bone to another.
c. False. Tendons are inelastic.
d. False. An aponeurosis is a sheet or fan-shaped tendon.
REF: Page 455

40.
a. False.
b. False.
c. False.
d. **Correct.**
REF: Page 456

41.
a. **Correct.**
b. False.
c. False.
d. False.
REF: Page 455, Figure 16.56 and Page 456

42.
a. False.
b. False.
c. **Correct.**
d. False.
REF: Page 456

43.
  a. False. Autoimmune disease in general, including MG, is more common in women than men
  b. **Correct.**
  c. False. In MG, acetylcholine release by the nerves supplying the muscle is normal, but autoantibodies have destroyed the receptors on the muscle to which acetylcholine needs to bind.
  d. False. Contraction of skeletal muscle becomes progressively weaker as they lose their ability to respond to acetylcholine, and they lose their tone and become flaccid.
  REF: Page 472

44.
  a. False.
  b. **Correct.** Iso = same, metric = length; in isometric contraction, as in attempting to pick up an immovable weight, the muscle is not able to shorten, so its tension increases.
  c. False. In isometric contraction, because the muscle is unable to shorten, the tension rises.
  d. False. The antagonistic muscle will relax.
  REF: Page 458

45.
  a. False.
  b. False.
  c. **Correct.**
  d. False.
  REF: Page 459

46.
  a. **Correct.**
  b. False.
  c. False.
  d. False.
  REF: Page 460, Figure 16.61

47.
  a. False.
  b. False.
  c. **Correct.**
  d. False.
  REF: Page 462, Figure 16.64

48.
  a. False. The biceps brachii mainly stabilises the shoulder joint, although it assists in elbow flexion.
  b. False. The flexor carpi radialis is a muscle of the forearm, which flexes the wrist.
  c. False. The triceps extends the elbow.
  d. **Correct.**
  REF: Page 464

49.
  a. False.
  b. False.
  c. False.
  d. **Correct.**
  REF: Page 465

50.
   a. False. The gastrocnemius overlies the soleus.
   b. False. The hamstrings (biceps femoris, semimembranous and semitendinosus) are thigh muscles, and the gastrocnemius forms the bulk of the calf.
   c. **Correct.**
   d. False. The sartorius is the longest muscle of the body.
   REF: Page 466

CHAPTER 17

Genetics

Feedback

1.
   a. False. Chromosomes contain the genes, but most DNA in the human cell is either apparently non-functional, or acts as start-stop signals for transcription.
   b. False. Alleles are different forms of the same gene, e.g. the tongue rolling gene has two forms, one that allows tongue rolling and one that does not.
   c. False. The genome refers to all the genetic material in a cell.
   d. **Correct.** Each gene codes for a different protein.
   REF: Page 475
2.
   a. False. There are 46 chromosomes in total, so only 23 pairs.
   b. False. The end regions are called telomeres, but they shorten with age and limit the number of times the cell can divide.
   c. **Correct.** The chromosome pairs are numbered starting with the largest.
   d. False. Chromosomes only form and become visible as the cell is preparing to divide.
   REF: Page 476
3.
   a. **Correct.**
   b. False. The sugar in DNA is always deoxyribose.
   c. False. Thiamine is a vitamin of the B complex; thymine is the similar sounding but chemically different base found in DNA.
   d. False. Uracil is not found in DNA, but is used to build RNA.
   REF: Page 477
4.
   a. False.
   b. **Correct.**
   c. False.
   d. False.
   REF: Page 477
5.
   a. False. Cri-du-chat is due to an incomplete chromosome 5.
   b. False. Phenylketonuria is due to a faulty gene on chromosome 12.
   c. **Correct.** Down's syndrome is due to an extra copy of chromosome 21.
   d. False. Cystic fibrosis is due to a faulty gene on chromosome 7.
   REF: Page 485

6.

    a. False. Uracil is used in RNA to replace thymine, so it always pairs with adenine.

    b. False. Cytosine pairs with guanine.

    c. False. Guanine pairs with cytosine, and uracil pairs with adenine.

    d. **Correct.**

REF: Page 477

7.

    a. **Correct.** The mitochondrial DNA codes mainly for enzymes involved in energy production, important to mitochondrial function.

    b. False.

    c. False.

    d. False.

REF: Page 477

8.

    a. False. mRNA is produced in the nucleus from DNA.

    b. False. Transcription of a gene produces mRNA.

    c. **Correct.**

    d. False. mRNA is produced as a result of gene activation.

REF: Page 478

9.

    a. False.

    b. **Correct.**

    c. False.

    d. False.

REF: Page 479

10.

    a. False.

    b. False.

    c. False.

    d. **Correct.** Haploid means half the normal genetic complement of a cell. Gametes (ova and spermatozoa) are haploid so that when one of each fuse to form a zygote, the new cell has the correct genetic complement.

REF: Page 480

11.

    a. False. Meiosis involves two distinct cell divisions.

    b. False. Quite the opposite: the function of meiosis is to mix up the genetic material during copying and division, so that the four daughter cells are different to each other and to the parent cell.

    c. **Correct.** The second cell division involves separation of the chromatids from the two daughter cells of the first division.

    d. False. Crossing over takes place during the first meiotic division.

REF: Page 480

12.

    a. False. The Tt genotype is heterozygous.

    b. False. tt is homozygous recessive.

    c. False. TT genotype, with two dominant forms of the gene, is tongue rolling.

    d. **Correct.** Either TT or Tt genotypes are tongue rollers, as they both have at least one copy of the dominant gene.

REF: Page 481

13.
    a. **Correct.**
    b. False.
    c. False.
    d. False.
    REF: Page 481

14.
    a. False.
    b. False.
    c. False.
    d. **Correct.** Heterozygous means that the two copies of the gene are different, one dominant and one recessive. If we use G (dominant form) and g (recessive form) for this, both parents therefore have genotype Gg. Do the Punnett square, and you see that half the children inherit two identical forms from their parents and two inherit one of each form. Thus, 50% are homozygous.
    REF: Page 482, Figure 17.9

15.
    a. False.
    b. **Correct.** Using G for the dominant gene and g for the recessive gene, the father is Gg and the mother is gg. Do the Punnett square, and the four possible combinations in the children are Gg, Gg, gg and gg.
    c. False.
    d. False.
    REF: Page 482

16.
    a. **Correct.** A child can only have blood group O if they inherit the recessive o gene from both parents. If a parent has blood group AB, this means that their genotype is AB, i.e., they have an A gene and a B gene, and no o gene; this mother could never have a child with blood group O, as she has no o gene to pass on. This father could potentially have a child with blood group O, as he must have two copies of the recessive o gene, but not with this mother.
    b, c and d. False. Parents with blood groups A or B may have genotype AA or Ao, or BB or Bo, so may be able to produce a child with blood group O; from the information here, it cannot be ruled out.
    REF: Page 482, Figure 17.10

17.
    a. False. Women inherit two copies of a sex-linked gene because the two X chromosomes are matched in size, each with a complete set of genes.
    b. False. Sex-linked genes are carried on the X chromosome.
    c. **Correct.** Because the Y chromosome contains only about 86 genes compared to the 2000 on the X chromosome, males have only one copy of most of the sex-linked genes.
    d. False. Sex-linked genes are transmitted by females on the X chromosome.
    REF: Page 482

18.
    a. **Correct.** All daughters of this couple will be carriers of the gene.
    b. False. All sons of this couple will have normal colour vision.
    c. False. Sons cannot be carriers, as a carrier has two copies of a gene, one of them the faulty gene; with sex linked genes, males only have one copy.
    d. False. All daughters will be heterozygous for the gene.
    REF: Pages 482 and 483

19.

    a. False. It is always the first step in development of cancer, but most mutated cells die or are destroyed before this can happen.

    b. False. Many mutations are repaired by intracellular enzymes.

    c. False. A cell with a mutation will pass this to the daughter cells when it divides; if the mutation occurs in a gamete, then it will be passed to children.

    d. **Correct.** One of the most important roles of the immune system, immunological surveillance, is in identifying and destroying abnormal body cells.

    REF: Page 477

20.

    a. False. Individuals with Klinefelter syndrome have genotype XXY, so are biologically male.

    b. False. This condition is not caused by a faulty gene, but by an additional X chromosome.

    c. **Correct.** The condition is associated with mild learning disability.

    d. False. The condition causes infertility.

    REF: Page 485

CHAPTER 18

The Reproductive System

Feedback

1.
    a. **Correct.** The vestibular glands, located immediately adjacent to the vaginal opening, produce secretions to keep the vulva moist.
    b. False. The cervix is internal.
    c. False. The perineum is the area between the anal opening and the base of the labia minora.
    d. False. The mons pubis is the fatty pad overlying the pubic bone.
    REF: Page 488

2.
    a. False.
    b. False.
    c. **Correct.**
    d. False.
    REF: Figure 18.2

3.
    a. **Correct.** The normal uterus is tilted forward (anteverted).
    b. False. The uterus is superior to the bladder.
    c. False. The uterus is anterior to the vesicouterine pouch.
    d. False. The uterus is anterior to the rectum.
    REF: Page 491, Figure 18.3

4.
    a. False. The posterior wall is longer than the anterior wall (see Fig. 18.3).
    b. False. The uterine cervix projects into its proximal end.
    c. **Correct.** It is kept moist by cervical secretions.
    d. False. The rugae (folds) of the vaginal wall allow the vagina to expand.
    REF: Page 490

5.
    a. False.
    b. False.
    c. False.
    d. **Correct.**
    REF: Page 491

6.
    a. False.
    b. **Correct.**
    c. False.
    d. False.
    REF: Figure 18.5

7.
   a. False.
   b. **Correct.**
   c. False.
   d. False.
   REF: Figure 18.5

8.
   a. **Correct.**
   b. False. This describes the broad ligament.
   c. False. This describes the uterosacral ligament.
   d. False. This describes the cardinal ligament.
   REF: Page 492, Figure 18.6

9.
   a. False.
   b. False.
   c. **Correct.**
   d. False.
   REF: Page 505

10.
   a. False.
   b. False.
   c. False.
   d. **Correct.**
   REF: Page 503

11.
   a. False. The fimbriae extend from the distal end of the uterine tubes.
   b. **Correct.**
   c. False. They form a trumpet-like structure at the distal end of the tubes.
   d. False. Fertilisation usually occurs within the uterine tubes.
   REF: Page 493

12.
   a. **Correct.**
   b. False. The mesovarium secures the ovary to the back of the broad ligament.
   c. False. The developing follicles, found in the cortex, secrete the female sex hormones.
   d. False. The medulla contains nerves, blood vessels and lymphatics.
   REF: Page 493

13.
   a. and b. False. The gonadotrophins are released by the anterior pituitary gland.
   c. **Correct.** In addition to luteinising hormone (LH), follicle stimulating hormone (FSH) is also a gonadotrophin.
   d. False.
   REF: Page 494, Figure 18.9

14.
   a. False. Progesterone is secreted in the second half of the cycle.
   b. False. FSH triggers follicle maturation, but not release.
   c. False. Oestrogen and progesterone are secreted together in the second half of the cycle.
   d. **Correct.** A pulse of LH (triggered by rising oestrogen) is released mid-cycle, and this triggers ovulation.
   REF: Page 495, Figure 18.10

15.
   a. False. The menstrual phase follows the secretory phase.
   b. **Correct.**
   c. False. FSH levels are low in the secretory phase to prevent further follicles developing.
   d. False. Follicular development is suppressed in the secretory phase.
   REF: Page 495, Figure 18.10

16.
   a. **Correct.** It is important that after ovulation, no further follicles develop in case this cycle results in pregnancy.
   b. False. High blood levels of oestrogen and progesterone together suppress the anterior pituitary, shutting down FSH and LH production.
   c. False. Under the influence of these two hormones in the second half of the cycle, the uterine lining becomes thickened, more vascular and secretory.
   d. False. High blood levels of oestrogen and progesterone together suppress the anterior pituitary, shutting down FSH and LH production. As LH maintains the corpus luteum, falling LH levels kills it.
   REF: Page 495

17.
   a. False.
   b. False.
   c. **Correct.**
   d. False.
   REF: Page 496

18.
   a. False.
   b. False.
   c. False.
   d. **Correct.**
   REF: Page 498

19.
   a. **Correct.**
   b. False.
   c. False.
   d. False.
   REF: Page 508

20.
   a. False.
   b. False.
   c. **Correct.** The testes, like the female ovaries, are the male gonads and produce the male gametes (spermatozoa).
   d. False.
   REF: Page 499

21.
   a. False.
   b. **Correct.**
   c. False.
   d. False.
   REF: Page 498, Figure 18.13 and Page 500

22.

    a. False.

    b. False.

    c. False.

    d. **Correct.**

    REF: Page 500

23.

    a. False.

    b. False.

    c. **Correct.**

    d. False.

    REF: Page 503, Figure 18.19

24.

    a. **Correct.**

    b. False. It is produced by the seminal vesicles.

    c. False. It is viscous.

    d. False. It is slightly alkaline to neutralise the acidity of the vagina.

    REF: Page 500

25.

    a. and c. False. Both apply to the corpora spongiosum, the central cylindrical mass of erectile tissue.

    b. **Correct.**

    d. False. The prepuce (foreskin) is a fold of skin enclosing the glans penis.

    REF: Page 501

26.

    a. False.

    b. False.

    c. **Correct.**

    d. False.

    REF: Page 501

27.

    a. False.

    b. False.

    c. False.

    d. **Correct.**

    REF: Page 503

28.

    a. False.

    b. **Correct.**

    c. False.

    d. False.

    REF: Page 509

29.

    a. **Correct.**

    b. False.

    c. False.

    d. False.

    REF: Page 504, Table 18.1

30.
    a. False.
    b. False.
    c. **Correct.**
    d. False.
    REF: Page 504, Table 18.1